STEEL CITY

Dedicated to the memory of Alan Fenton-Smith, who was a constant source of encouragement no matter how stormy the sea. Sheffield's loss is heaven's gain.

And to Peter Furnell, whose calm patience in any circumstance over many decades continues to be inspirational.

STEEL CITY PRESS

This first edition published in 2022 by Steel City Press, 9 Ravenscroft Close, Sheffield, S13 8PN.
Website: www.steelcitypress.co.uk

Where's God When I'm Depressed?
ISBN 978-1-913047-34-4

Copyright © 2022 Jonathan Arnott

All rights reserved. This book or any portion thereof may not be reproduced or used in any manner whatsoever without the express written permission of the publisher except for the use of brief quotations in a book review.

All Scripture quotations, unless otherwise indicated, are taken from the Holy Bible, New International Version®, NIV®. Copyright ©1973, 1978, 1984, 2011 by Biblica, Inc.™ Used by permission of Zondervan. All rights reserved worldwide. www.zondervan.com. The "NIV" and "New International Version" are trademarks registered in the United States Patent and Trademark Office by Biblica, Inc.™

CONTENTS

Introduction	Page 5
Chapter 1: The juniper tree	Page 9
Chapter 2: It's not a sin to be depressed...	Page 14
Chapter 3: ...But don't let depression lead to sin	Page 22
Chapter 4: God loves you. Unconditionally.	Page 28
Chapter 5: You're never 'not good enough' for God	Page 33
Chapter 6: Father God	Page 40
Chapter 7: The problem of suffering	Page 44
Chapter 8: In the world but not of it	Page 52
Chapter 9: Guilt and forgiveness	Page 61
Chapter 10: Testing times	Page 67
Chapter 11: Raise a hallelujah	Page 78
Chapter 12: A higher purpose	Page 83
Chapter 13: Practical advice	Page 88

Introduction

"He heals the brokenhearted and binds up their wounds"
- Psalm 147:3

Depression hurts. I mean that literally. For me, when I'm depressed my arms and legs ache (think of the muscle pains you get with a nasty cold or a flu). My energy levels drop, to the point that even getting out of bed is a physical struggle as well as a mental one. The tiniest noise will set me off. Someone in the same room is eating, and I hear every crunch. The world feels too loud. I want to be alone, but if I'm alone I feel lonely and want to be around people. Sometimes it'll stop me sleeping, leaving me still awake at 5am. Depression causes insomnia. Insomnia causes depression.

And in the midst of all this, maybe a wonderful friend (Christian or not) will offer advice. "Have you tried...", they suggest helpfully, and then come up with ideas that I've heard over and over again for decades and tried many times in the past. I want to be grateful, to be thankful that they care, but instead it makes me more frustrated than I was before. I feel that there must be something 'different' about me, because those well-meaning ideas seem to work for everyone else. For normal people. Maybe I'm not normal...

Do you see how things can spiral out of control? Nothing is logical. Nothing makes sense. The whole thing goes round in a vicious circle that won't break itself. Someone who doesn't understand depression will eventually run out of ideas, and that's when they suggest 'tablets'. Now, I'm not saying that there aren't situations in which medication can help as part of an overall package of treatment. They're not an easy answer either. They have side effects, and then getting off them again can cause withdrawal symptoms. In the first couple of weeks, whilst the body is getting used to the new medication, the depression can get worse before it gets better. There's always a question of whether the benefits outweigh the problems. If, after prayer and consultation with your doctor, it seems that taking medication is the right decision, then I would be fully supportive of that decision. But if it's just a friend who's feeling like the only thing left in their head to suggest is 'tablets', there's a problem. And often it'll be the closest friends to you, the ones you speak to on a regular basis, the ones you trust the most, who will be suggesting anything that they think might make you feel better. It comes from the right heart, but it doesn't mean that it's helpful.

I'm writing this book for two main reasons. If you don't have depression, I want you to understand a bit more about it so that you're able to help others. People who don't suffer with depression find it difficult to comprehend what's actually going on when someone is depressed. They feel lost because they don't understand the mindset. And to be fair, how could they understand when they haven't experienced it themselves?

If you do have depression, everyone is different but one of the most common feelings is "nobody understands me". I don't want to convince you that I understand you (although I'll try my best). I'm not perfect. I know that. As a Christian, of course it's part of my DNA to be there and try to help. More importantly, I want you to know that God understands what you're going through. To understand that it is heartbreaking for Him to see you heartbroken. That He is fully able to sympathise with what we're going through because Jesus went through every kind of test and trial himself (Hebrews 4). I want you to understand that no matter how you are feeling, His overwhelming love for you is always there. It never changes, never fails. When everything else around you feels like it's going wrong, God's love is as solid as a rock.

This is, I think, the fifth time that I've sat down to try to write this book. Sometimes when circumstances seem to conspire to prevent you following what you believe is of God, that can be an indication that it's worth double-checking whether you're sure that it's definitely what you're supposed to be doing. But in this case, what happened on each of the other four times has shown me very much that this is needed.

The first time I tried to write, I got a few words onto my computer screen before a friend who suffers with depression told me about an issue with a relationship. I put the computer down and helped as best as I could. The second time, I tried writing late in the evening. I got a phone call from a friend at the other end of the country, crying her eyes out going through a mental health crisis. I tried a third time the next day to start writing, and then another friend phoned needing support because he thought he'd seriously messed up a situation in his own life. Then, the fourth time, I was just starting to write just after midnight when I heard loud footsteps coming down the stairs.

I rushed through to the kitchen to see what was happening. A friend who suffers from depression and was staying over for a few days had headed over to the kitchen and was hiding a pair of meat scissors behind her back. Rather than let me help, she rushed into a corner and turned away from me. What could I do? There wasn't time to talk through things. I couldn't even wrestle the scissors away: that would have risked accidentally causing a far more serious injury. And then I heard the sound of scissors cutting into flesh.

Difficult, isn't it? Wouldn't you also be heartbroken in that moment, caring for a Christian who's struggling so much that they've felt the only way of getting some temporary relief was through self-harm.

We talked. We prayed. I felt grieved in my spirit to see that happen, but I remembered that Jesus in His ministry simply met people where they were at. I took my friend to clean up the wounds. Isn't that what God does? He "heals the brokenhearted and binds up their wounds". Aren't we as Christians called to follow His example, to be "imitators of God" (Ephesians 5)? That situation was a physical manifestation of deep hurt inside.

I don't need to tell you, at least right now, any more of that situation. But each of those four situations confirmed something for me: that there is a real need to write this book. There's an epidemic of depression throughout Western society. Christians don't have immunity to it, but we do have more tools in our toolbox when it comes to responding to those feelings. We have prayer, we have worship, we have fellowship. More importantly, we have the knowledge that we are safe within God's arms.

Chapter 1

"I have had enough, Lord," he said. "Take my life; I am no better than my ancestors." Then he lay down under the bush and fell asleep. - 1 Kings 19:4-5

Elijah is sitting under the juniper tree. He is, to use the modern word, depressed - to the point that he asks God to kill him. I don't get the sense, reading that passage in 1 Kings 19, that it's even just a passing 'cry for help'. It seems that Elijah has come to the end of his tether. He's got a high-profile job as a prophet of God. All he's done is follow God's direction, and he's been rushing from place to place. Jezebel has vowed to kill him. Elijah is exhausted physically, mentally and spiritually. He sits under the juniper tree [white broom tree] and prays for his life to end.

But even as Elijah does this, God is already helping. The juniper tree is symbolic in the Bible as a place of safety, a refuge from the heat. Its shade is useful for desert travellers wanting to avoid the harsh sun beating down on their heads. Under the juniper tree, Elijah is already receiving God's protection. Elijah falls asleep.

I read an article recently online, which I'm sure was well-meaning. It said that so many Christians 'choose' to sit under the juniper tree in a wilderness of despair and depression. Harsh words, words which could almost come across as 'blaming' Christians for being depressed. I don't want to be overly critical either, because there certainly is an element of truth in the idea that Christians should see the positives when we have Christ and His Holy Spirit living within us. But that's really not the way to deal with someone who's suffering from depression.

How did God deal with Elijah? Would God have a go at Elijah for not having enough faith? Elijah had seen God's faithfulness through miracles and now, in his time of depression, he was starting to assume that God wouldn't be faithful again. I can imagine that many Christians would 'secretly' want to shout at Elijah and tell him to wake up to the amazing things that God was doing. If only we could see such miracles in our own lives!

No. God doesn't do that. He provides Elijah with shade. He provides Elijah with rest. He provides Elijah with food. He provides Elijah with drink. He sends an angel to provide the nourishment and sustenance that Elijah will need to continue his journey.

Jokingly, I might say that all Elijah really needed was food and a nap. That's actually not so far from the truth: when suffering from depression, meeting the basic physical needs can help. If you're hungry, tired, overheating and thirsty then the world's problems probably do seem a bit worse than they actually are. God takes care of all those things for Elijah, and there is something miraculous about the way in which it all happens.

God simply met Elijah where he was at and helped him. No negativity, no criticism, just simple practical caring. It's such a basic lesson for when you're caring for someone who's depressed. You'd be surprised how often food plays a major role - because it meets a physical need, but also because it's part of a process of fellowship.

Over the years, spending time with friends who are struggling has often involved that. We'd make white chocolate truffles together, or I'd take them out for a meal. I've lost count of the number of times I've cooked midnight pancakes. It's a principle I've extended to other situations in life. Nine times out of ten if I'm meeting someone for a chat or a work meeting, I try to do so over lunch. If there's a difficult conversation that needs having, why not buy someone food whilst you're doing it?

If you're feeling depressed, making sure that you've had enough to eat and drink is an important form of self-care. There's a moment of 'I can't even be bothered to make myself something to eat' which is probably one of the most important feelings that you should fight. You're going to need that nourishment to be able to face the day.

No matter what happens, God is *never going to abandon you*. He loves you in the most incredible way. When you go wrong, He won't. When you're feeling so down that you don't even know what you really need, He provides it for you. Elijah asked God to kill him. God could have answered that prayer, and we would never have heard anything more of Elijah. But He didn't. He knew what Elijah needed, even though Elijah didn't know himself.

God knows you better than you know yourself: *"Indeed, the very hairs of your head are all numbered. Don't be afraid; you are worth more than many sparrows."* - Luke 12:7. I don't think Luke is meaning that figuratively. God actually knows every single hair on your head, every line on your fingerprint, every up and down in your life, and every worry that seems so insignificant during the day but becomes paralysingly bad when you wake up at 3am in a panic.

When you're depressed, there are many of the Psalms which speak on this point. It's not a surprise, is it? Psalms were meant to be sung. They're songs of praise and worship to God. They're also real and down-to-earth: real situations, real problem and real encouragement. I love Psalm 139 when it comes to showing how well God knows us:

"You have searched me, Lord, and you know me. You know when I sit and when I rise; you perceive my thoughts from afar.

You discern my going out and my lying down; you are familiar with all my ways. Before a word is on my tongue you, Lord, know it completely.

You hem me in behind and before, and you lay your hand upon me. Such knowledge is too wonderful for me, too lofty for me to attain.

Where can I go from your Spirit? Where can I flee from your presence? If I go up to the heavens, you are there; if I make my bed in the depths, you are there.

If I rise on the wings of the dawn, if I settle on the far side of the sea, even there your hand will guide me, your right hand will hold me fast.

If I say, "Surely the darkness will hide me and the light become night around me," even the darkness will not be dark to you; the night will shine like the day, for darkness is as light to you.

For you created my inmost being; you knit me together in my mother's womb. I praise you because I am fearfully and wonderfully made; your works are wonderful, I know that full well.

My frame was not hidden from you when I was made in the secret place, when I was woven together in the depths of the earth. Your eyes saw my unformed body; all the days ordained for me were written in your book before one of them came to be.

How precious to me are your thoughts, God! How vast is the sum of them! Were I to count them, they would outnumber the grains of sand - when I awake, I am still with you." - Psalm 139: 1-18

Wow! God knows everything about us. He knows our thoughts, understands whatever we're going through. He knows us in such detail that even as our bodies were being formed before birth, He knew every little detail. You know that by just 12 weeks of pregnancy, 26 weeks before the baby is born, it already has a heartbeat, electrical brain activity, and even fingerprints and fingernails? Doctors can see those things through ultrasound scans but God just knows every single detail. He knew every little detail about you not just 26 weeks (6 months) before you were born but right from the very first day that you were conceived. And He is there. He is there to protect you. That might feel difficult to believe sometimes, and that's not even a lack of faith but a symptom of depression. When everything around you feels like your world is falling apart, how do you believe in something that seems just too good to be true?

Humans are going to fail you. I try my best, but I'll fail from time to time. As someone who suffers from depression myself, sometimes it's tough when I'm caring for other people who are going through the same thing. It's exhausting and I'm not always going to respond in the right way 100% of the time. And you're going to fail from time to time too; however much it's right to do your best in every situation, just understand that God doesn't expect absolute perfection from you either.

Chapter 2 -
It's not a sin to be depressed...

"Someone who is struggling with depression might also be sinning or be the victim of another person's sin, but depression isn't a sin. It is the outcome of sin. It is the result of another's sin. In and of itself though, depression is not the problem. It is the response to the problem."

- Mercy Multiplied

In the Bible, it might be fair to say that God didn't like people moaning at Him. He wasn't impressed by the Israelites seeing every possible problem with the Promised Land. He didn't like complaints which stemmed simply from a lack of faith. I guess that is probably why so many Christians can have a problem with helping others through depression: they see depression as though it's just the same as the moaning of an ungrateful people or the disciples not having enough faith despite Jesus being physically right there with them.

I mean, those things are certainly sinful. But - and I can't stress this enough - **that's not what depression is.** In the last chapter we saw that God went out of His way to look after Elijah when he was in despair. Psalm 18:6 tells us that *"In my distress I called to the LORD; I cried to my God for help. From his temple he heard my voice; my cry came before him, into his ears"*. When we're distressed, God is right there with us. He's described as our 'refuge' and our 'strength'. And if you think Elijah was struggling, just listen to what Jeremiah said: *"Cursed be the day I was born"* (Jeremiah 20:14) and *"Why did I ever come out of the womb to see trouble and sorrow and to end my days in shame?"* (Jeremiah 20:18).

Have you ever felt like that? That self-hatred or just wishing that it would 'all end', even if that doesn't mean suicidal thoughts or tendencies but just a real feeling that you've reached the end of your tether and you can't see a way out? As you can't 'see' a way out, there's a feeling of being trapped. If you don't believe that there's any way things can get better, it's even difficult to do the basics: I know I've had many times in the past when I can't bring myself to pray about something because it feels like it will only feel even more hopeless. That's not a reaction in a 'normal' situation: there are many times that I can, and do, pray in faith as well. Maybe there's a difference between 'me' and 'other people': that is, I can pray for other people going through tough situations even when I'm depressed. When it's about myself, I find that more tricky. In that sense I feel as though I can identify with Jeremiah's feelings.

In this situation I feel that Jeremiah is in despair, but there's a difference between Jeremiah and Elijah. Elijah was exhausted physically, mentally and emotionally and fleeing for his life. The impression I get from Jeremiah is different, more of a meltdown. It's a situation where everything has got on top of him and he maybe just needs some space to calm down. What does God do? Does He have a go at Jeremiah? No. Does He intervene like He did with Elijah? No, not that either. I get the impression that Jeremiah's words are spoken from a position of despair, and he's exaggerating because of how he feels at the time. Instead, we don't read of any response from God: Jeremiah is given the space he needs to get everything out of his system.

But despite Jeremiah's sadness, we see by chapter 29 that his words become more encouraging. You probably know one of the most famous verses of the Bible: *"For I know the plans I have for you," declares the Lord, "plans to prosper you and not to harm you, plans to give you hope and a future"* - Jeremiah 29:11. We lift that verse out of its context and talk about how amazing it is that God has a hope and a future for us. How many times, though, do we bother to look even one verse before? The phrase 'when seventy years are done' is quite important in this context: God has plans for us, amazing plans, but that doesn't mean that we won't be waiting for a long time. It's not our timing but His timing that matters, however frustrating that might be.

In Jeremiah 31:1 we read the promise that speaks of that restoration between God and his people: *"At that time...I will be the God of all the families of Israel, and they will be my people"*. That sounds great, doesn't it? All sweetness and happiness. But then comes one of the most difficult verses in the Bible.

I don't want to hide from this. The verse shakes me to my core every time I read it. When I was in Jerusalem, I found the Holocaust Memorial Museum by accident: I just happened to be walking past it (long story why that happened, but I'm sure that God was a part of it all) and decided to go in. I saw some horrific things, understanding the terrors which the Nazis had inflicted on people just for being Jewish. I can't even begin to describe the grief that I felt, seeing example after example of how human beings had been treated as worse than animals by sadistic guards on an industrial scale. One memory sticks with me more than any other. Jewish people are urged to treat the Old Testament with respect. They wouldn't put a Bible on the floor, for example. So when I saw how a Jewish tailor had been forced against his will to sew Bible passages into a suit, and seeing the stains of his blood which had dripped onto that suit, it filled me with horror. I can't even begin to process my feelings about how evil and depraved those actions were, with absolutely no reason whatsoever.

It showed the evil of the Nazis, the way they had persecuted and killed millions of Jewish people. Generations later, the Jewish people still feel the pain and trauma of what happened to them at that time. And then, in the centre of the room, stood a Bible verse. From the *same chapter* as that beautiful promise I just quoted.

"A voice is heard in Ramah, mourning and great weeping, Rachel weeping for her children and refusing to be comforted, because they are no more." - Jeremiah 31:15

I'll never forget that Bible verse. Rachel here is symbolic: all the way back in Genesis, Jacob and Rachel were the parents of Joseph (think: amazing technicolour dreamcoat). The reference to Rachel's children is talking about her descendants, which means so much more in Jewish culture than it does in Western nations. A lot of Biblical prophecies can be true in more than one way: here it refers both to the situation in Jeremiah, and, in the hearts and minds of the Jewish people, also to the horrors of the Holocaust.

We can't even begin to imagine those levels of grief. The reason I'm talking about this is that the kind of sadness that reaches right into your very soul is something which is known and understood in the Bible. How could Rachel be comforted? What could anybody possibly say to help her to feel better? And yet, there's a promise attached. It's a promise which is true both at the time (to Jeremiah) and in the longer term to the whole nation of Israel. It's a promise that the Jewish people will return to their own land. Jeremiah 31:16-17 goes on to say:

Restrain your voice from weeping and your eyes from tears, for your work will be rewarded," declares the Lord. "They will return from the land of the enemy. So there is hope for your descendants," declares the Lord. "Your children will return to their own land."

As human beings, we're naturally going to 'see' things in terms of the physical world. But the few years we're on this planet are only a tiny speck in comparison with the 'forever', the eternal existence that we'll have together with God. We'll talk about this more in the chapter on suffering, but for now I'll just say that there is always a longer-term plan and there is always hope. The nation of Israel has indeed been restored. After nearly two thousand years of being scattered all over the world after the Romans kicked them out of their country, they finally have their own land once again.

Are you sad? It's okay to be sad. Are you depressed? It's okay to be depressed. But don't ever lose sight of the fact that God is there right with you, no matter what. Whatever your despair, when you cry God 'cries with you'.

I've seen, so many times, Christians who are depressed go into a spiral. Here's how the thinking goes:

The Bible talks about joy, over and over again.

I don't feel joy. I feel sad.

Why don't I feel that joy?

What's wrong with me?

Am I doing something wrong?

Is this my fault?

Am I sinning?

Nobody else is depressed.

Everyone else seems to be happy.

I've prayed about this. I'm still depressed.

Maybe God has abandoned me...

Do you see how that thought process spirals out of control so quickly? That's why it can be so toxic when anyone tries to tell you that depression is sinful, or shows you an inspirational Bible verse as though it's going to be a quick-fix for what you're going through.

Compare that to how God responds in the Bible. He is a caregiver, providing Elijah and Jeremiah with what they both need in their own individual situations. He doesn't challenge the sad feelings directly, but helps by doing the things that are needed to build them up. I think that's a great model for how to help someone who is depressed. Remember I talked about cooking midnight pancakes for a friend suffering from depression? Or the times (and it's happened with more than one person) when I've had to care for someone who's self-harmed, helping them to clean up their wounds afterwards. Those simple acts of kindness can often speak much more than anything you could actually *say* about their situation. Does someone need sleep? Give them a comfy bed for the night. Do they need to cry? Give them a shoulder to cry on.

If there's one thing you need when looking after someone who's depressed, it's patience. You see how that thinking spiralled out of control? Depression does that. When someone is depressed, they're not thinking logically. They've reinforced the negatives, time after time after time, in their head. A few kind words aren't going to change that. It's a slow process, being there for them. Fortunately, as Christians, we should have the 'fruits of the spirit' mentioned in Galatians 5:22-23:

"But the fruit of the Spirit is love, joy, peace, forbearance [patience], kindness, goodness, faithfulness, gentleness and self-control"

We've already talked a little about joy, but each of the others are naturally exactly what someone who is suffering from depression needs from you. They need you to show them love (i.e. a reflection of God's love for them). If you are able to remain peaceful, calm during their storm, you can help to provide that foundation. You'll need to be patient because this isn't something that is likely to be completely cured with a single prayer (though God can heal people of depression), and the causes of this particular depressive state might seem trivial to you. Someone who has been broken by the nastiness within the world needs your kindness, goodness and faithfulness: maybe they've been abandoned time and time again; if you simply show them that you're going to stick around and that you're there, it makes a huge difference. Then there is self-control. Depression is not easy for others to deal with. Sometimes you might get that urge to tell someone to just 'snap out of it', or words to that effect. Self-control is so important.

Is one of your friends or family members depressed? Test your response against Galatians 5. Do you match up to that? If not, you know what you need to do to help them. The good part is that those things naturally flow from having the Holy Spirit inside you; the bad part is that your own sinful nature rebels against such things.

Isaiah 42:3 says *"A bruised reed he will not break, and a smouldering wick he will not snuff out"*. Those words speak to God's compassion. He understands what someone is going through: that's another reason I say it is not a sin to be depressed. God's response when you're bruised or when your fire has been reduced to burning embers is not to do anything to make the situation worse. He doesn't criticise the reed for being bruised, or the wick because it's only smouldering.

In fact, the ancient Hebrew word translated as 'bruised' means far more than what we think of it as. It implies a deep hurt, a level of internal damage that is crippling. It's more like internal bleeding or trauma to an organ, and yet that hurt might not be immediately visible to everyone around you.

I recognise that description: it's a deep kind of hurt, and God's overwhelming care is to say - in essence - that He won't let things go too far. He's your safety net. That's the promise: however bad things get, He is still right there for you in your time of need. We see the same principle in 1 Corinthians 10:13:

"No temptation has overtaken you except what is common to mankind. And God is faithful; he will not let you be tempted beyond what you can bear. But when you are tempted, he will also provide a way out so that you can endure it."

But how does 'tempted' relate to depression? You might think that's about sin, surely? The thing is, that word can also be translated as 'tested': no matter how you're tested in life, God will always be faithful. And the most testing times, more than anything else, are those when depression flares up. There will always be a way out, and that's a promise!

Don't ever think that it's a sin to be depressed. God cares more than you could possibly understand or imagine.

"Now to him who is able to do immeasurably more than all we ask or imagine, according to his power that is at work within us, to him be glory in the church and in Christ Jesus throughout all generations, for ever and ever! Amen." - Ephesians 3: 20-21

Chapter 3 -
...but depression can lead to sin

He told them another parable: "The kingdom of heaven is like a mustard seed, which a man took and planted in his field. Though it is the smallest of all seeds, yet when it grows, it is the largest of garden plants and becomes a tree, so that the birds come and perch in its branches."

- Matthew 13:31-32

I know. This chapter title isn't easy. You probably don't want to hear it. It's encouraging though, honest! I want you to think about the widow in Mark 12: 41-44, who gave everything she had even though it was a tiny amount of money:

"Jesus sat down opposite the place where the offerings were put and watched the crowd putting their money into the temple treasury. Many rich people threw in large amounts. But a poor widow came and put in two very small copper coins, worth only a few cents.

Calling his disciples to him, Jesus said, "Truly I tell you, this poor widow has put more into the treasury than all the others. They all gave out of their wealth; but she, out of her poverty, put in everything—all she had to live on.""

Can you imagine how much of a show those rich people were putting on when they donated huge amounts to the temple? If so, they were the ones doing the sinning. Jesus had just been warning about that kind of arrogance earlier in the chapter. Matthew 6 tells us *"So when you give to the needy, do not announce it with trumpets, as the hypocrites do in the synagogues and on the streets, to be honored by others. Truly I tell you, they have received their reward in full. But when you give to the needy, do not let your left hand know what your right hand is doing, so that your giving may be in secret. Then your Father, who sees what is done in secret, will reward you."* People can boast about the things they do for God, trying to make themselves sound like some kind of super-Christian. People in leadership can so easily fall into that self-centred trap, but I can honestly hand-on-heart say that hasn't applied to anyone who's been in leadership at any church I've attended regularly over the last decade or two. In fact, the leaders have been some of the most wonderful, down-to-earth, humble people you could ever possibly hope to meet. In 2 Corinthians 11, Paul warns about the potential arrogance from so-called 'super-apostles'. Ask yourself the question: is that leader signposting God, or signposting themselves? I'm fortunate that the answer has been 'God' in my direct experience, but I've seen examples of the opposite too. That's not what God cares about. God doesn't care whether you're an amazing public speaker. He's not fussed whether you have a beautiful turn of phrase, whether you can write a wonderful book. He doesn't care whether you're capable of playing the most beautiful of music, or if you can make a room sparkle with your wit and humour. He cares only that you give what you are able to give, and in the right spirit.

When you're feeling down and broken, does God expect the same of you that He would expect of someone whose life is all going perfectly? No - in just the same way that nobody would expect someone suffering from flu to be able to run a marathon. God understood that the widow who could only give a couple of cents was giving everything that she had. The Bible (think of the Parable of the Talents) sometimes uses money as a metaphor for ability. The widow's tiny offering isn't just about money, it's about our heart attitude towards God. Maybe when you're depressed you are physically and emotionally exhausted. You feel like you haven't got very much that you can 'give' back to other people. That's okay. God never asks more than you're capable of. But even if it's only a tiny amount, God still wants you to do what you can through that time of depression.

Depression isn't a sin. Of course it isn't. And God will richly bless you for just doing the little bits of helping others that you're able to do. It doesn't need to be 50-50 in every situation in life, every friendship. Maybe others are supporting you right now more than you're supporting them, and that's okay: the Bible tells us to put other people first. If someone is putting you first, then that's them being obedient to God and it's fantastic that they care enough to do that for you. But even in those times, you can still - in small ways - simply do the things that you can do for Him.

Sometimes your depression might be so overpowering and overwhelming that there really isn't much at all that you can do. One of my favourite Bible verses is at the beginning of the passage about putting on the armour of God - Ephesians 6: 13. *"Therefore put on the full armour of God, so that when the day of evil comes, you may be able to stand your ground, **and after you have done everything**, to stand."* That phrase 'after you have done everything' gets me every time. In life everything will be thrown at us. We have God, and we have an enemy who will do anything to stop us. Our enemy will attempt to derail us by any possible means, and we stand our ground.

Then comes the 'after you have done everything'. You've fought against it with all your might. You've resisted the devil's schemes and you've expended almost every last drop of energy just making it through the day. You're at the end of your tether. You've done everything. And then, there's the 'afterwards'. After you've done everything. It's the calm after the storm. You have zero energy left. And still, after that, you stand. In defiance. No matter how you feel, you still remain faithful to God. You're still standing. Nobody is ever going to stop you. That's amazing!

So how could depression lead to sin? Well, you know that 'little' thing that you're capable of? The thing that seems so tiny and insignificant? The thing you worry other people will think is pathetic, or that they'll laugh at you because that's the only thing you've got to offer? That. Isn't it so abundantly precious to God? That's your 'widow's mite'. Jesus said that widow had given more into the Treasury than everyone else. He sees your 'two cents' as more valuable than someone else's hundreds of pounds, because your emotional 'two cents' is everything that you had to give.

It's so easy, isn't it, to devalue the little tiny things that you can do? So easy to just...not...because they seem like they couldn't possibly be of any use to anybody. You start joining in with the people you imagine would laugh at you and...well, suddenly you're into a trap. When you do nothing at all, that 'nothing' can become a prison.

I think that matters for another reason too. Zechariah 4:10 (NIV) us "*Who dares despise the day of small things?*" and the New Living Translation then explains that the Lord rejoices to see the work begin. (*Note: I'm switching translations there because the NIV version is more complex and mixes the same sentiment into the next concept*). Remember that mustard seed at the start of the chapter? It grew into a huge tree. David had just five stones in his sling, but it was enough to save his nation from Goliath and an opposing army. In John 6, Jesus turned five small loaves of bread and two fish into a feast for five thousand people, with baskets more left over. From something small came abundance because God was at the centre. God could take something little and turn it into something incredible.

God asks only that you do what you can, according to your ability. He never puts you under a burden that you can't bear. He asks only that you do what you can, and even if you can't do so much when you're depressed, He simply wants you to obey in those little ways. And who knows? Those small things might well explode into something far bigger.

Sometimes the root cause of depression can be a feeling of uselessness. Just overcoming that little mental hurdle, doing that one little thing, might give you the confidence to do another. And then another. And then maybe you start to recognise that it is actually getting somewhere, that you are actually making a difference. Suddenly, you feel that sense of purpose. You have a vision for something that you want to achieve, and…well, has your depression gone away? Probably not. But now there's something positive as well, a feeling that things maybe aren't hopeless. Romans 5:5 tells us that *"hope does not disappoint us, because God has poured out his love into our hearts by the Holy Spirit, whom he has given us."* Maybe a slightly different context for the word 'hope' there, but there's definitely a spiritual sense in which hope and expectation are intertwined: indeed, in many languages there is only one word which means both 'hope' and 'expect' at the same time. The word 'hope' means something more in the Bible than it seems at first glance in English.

Having some hope and a vision won't have cured your depression, but you might start to see a light at the end of the tunnel. You always had a purpose in God, but maybe that purpose starts to feel more real. Where there is no vision, the Proverb tells us, the people perish. It's hard-wired into us that we need to have something to look forward to, something to aim towards. Perhaps that's why there's evidence that people who won millions of pounds on the lottery end up being more sad than they were before. People who see 'money' as being a goal might realise that, once they have achieved that goal, it doesn't bring them happiness at all. Now that they have no goal, nothing to work towards, they find themselves lost. Money was always going to be a false friend, and now where is their hope?

False hope disappoints. Real hope, the hope that's rooted in Jesus Christ? That never disappoints us, as we saw in Romans 5. In the verse before, we're told that 'suffering' produces 'perseverance'. That sounds right: if we have faith in God, it should help us to keep going even through times of suffering - times of depression - even if 'keeping going' is just about the most you can possibly manage to do at the time. Then 'perseverance' produces 'character'. Yes, there's something about keeping going when things get tough that really develops us. And 'character' produces 'hope', which also makes sense if you think about it: you start to see the possibilities for how things can get better. Then, from those foundations, comes the consequence: that hope will not disappoint us. No matter what. Because in that sense, the hope comes from God rather than ourselves.

So can depression lead to sin? Yes, I think it can, but only if you allow it to. All that God needs from you, in this context, is a willingness to just do the things that you can. I said earlier that nobody would expect someone with flu to run a marathon. What if, instead, the athlete had broken a leg? They wouldn't be running a marathon but the doctors would be encouraging them to do exercises to maintain and build up their strength during the time of healing. Those simple exercises might seem like nothing, but they're vital components of the process of recovery.

Chapter 4 -
God loves you. Unconditionally.

"I asked Jesus, 'How much do you love me?' And Jesus said, 'This much.' Then He stretched out His arms and died."

David Wilkerson heard about the gang-based violence in New York. He believed that God was calling him to go and preach to gangs of teenagers on the streets. And so he went. He spoke to Nicky Cruz, the leader of the Mau Maus, telling him about God's love.

"You come near me and I'll kill you!", said Nicky Cruz.

"Yeah, you could do that", replied David Wilkerson. *"You could cut me up into a thousand pieces and lay them in the street, and every piece will still love you."*

Twice, Wilkerson spoke to Cruz. Twice, Cruz hit him. Nicky Cruz was saved at a later meeting, becoming an evangelist and director of the Teen Challenge programme in New York. Love. God's love for someone who thought nothing of taking out a knife and stabbing an enemy. No matter what was being done by Nicky Cruz or the Mau Mau gang, David Wilkerson had the courage to speak the truth. God loves you.

What bravery David Wilkerson showed! I would love to think that, in the same situation, I would be just as brave. And maybe, if God had spoken to me so clearly, I might manage to be just as obedient. Or not. But that's not the point I'm making right now. Look at God's compassion for Nicky Cruz. He was a gang leader, a criminal. The kind of person who would make you feel terrified if you saw him on the streets. Other gangs wanted him to die. The general public were scared of people like him. The police wanted him to be locked up so that he couldn't do any further harm to the community around him. And God? Well...God loved him. No matter what. Because God doesn't see the imperfections of who we are, no matter how bad they might be. God sees the potential. And whatever we've done in the past (an idea we'll come back to in the chapter on guilt), there is absolutely nothing which can't be wiped away by Christ's sacrifice for us on the cross.

"Very rarely will anyone die for a righteous man, though for a good man someone might possibly dare to die. But God demonstrates his own love for us in this: While we were still sinners, Christ died for us." - Romans 5: 7-8

What love! I know this is basic Bible stuff, but it's so important that it needs to be repeated. Maybe when you're feeling depressed, you might ask a question like 'how could God (or anyone) possibly love someone like me?'. Now whatever you've done, I bet it wasn't worse than Nicky Cruz. And God almost literally sent out a search party to find Nicky Cruz! I bet it wasn't worse than the Apostle Paul, who made it his life's mission to persecute and kill Christians - until God showed him the reality of what he was actually doing.

Do you accept that God loves everyone else?

*Do you accept that God loves **you**?*

When depressed, it's very easy to end up with a bit of 'cognitive dissonance' going on. You can answer the first question 'yes', and the second question 'no', without ever pausing for a moment to consider just how irrational that actually is. If God loves everyone else, what could possibly be so specially terrible about you that would mean you're the only exception who ever lived?

The phrase 'cognitive dissonance' refers to the habit of human beings to believe two things at the same time which contradict each other. Imagine you're on a diet. You think that you're just going to eat that bar of chocolate, because you're going to the gym later and you'll burn off those calories. Then, later, maybe you don't actually go to the gym. Or maybe you do go to the gym, and then you decide to 'reward' yourself by eating a couple of doughnuts. Instead of recognising that you're breaking the diet, you create a narrative in your own mind. You make yourself believe that you're following the diet...and then later, after following this logic for a few weeks, you wonder why you've not actually lost any weight. That's cognitive dissonance. The human brain loves to avoid being challenged, and so it's very easy for us to be a bit hypocritical with ourselves.

The kind of cognitive dissonance that you get when you're depressed is the oppositive. Instead of presenting things in the best possible light for yourself, like the person who considers chocolate to be a key part of their weight loss apparently (well isn't a cocoa bean a vegetable?), depression leads us to present everything in the worst possible light for ourselves.

That's where, in psychiatry, Cognitive Behavioural Therapy comes in. It tries to 'train' your brain to understand when your thought processes are in conflict with reality. Here's one exercise which could be used:

> **Take The Thought To Court: When you have a negative feeling, write down two lists:**
>
> **1. What is the evidence in favour of it?**
> **2. What is the evidence against it?**
>
> **Force yourself to decide whether that feeling is really true, or whether it's just your mind playing tricks on you. After a while, hopefully it becomes easier to recognise that those negative thoughts aren't actually accurate.**

It's also perfectly okay to apply a technique like 'Take the thought to court' to Christian situations. What evidence do you have to support your feeling when it comes to God? What evidence do you have against? And - thirdly - we can add something else as Christians: *What does the Bible say about it?*

If you trust in medical professionals about your mental health, but ignore God, then you're missing out on His power. It's like trying to use a toy with no batteries in. It's missing the thing that really makes it work.

If you trust in God, but don't want to listen to medical professionals, well, why do you think those medical professionals are there? The Bible tells us that *"The authorities that exist have been established by God"* (Romans 13:1). God's provision for you includes His provision of doctors and nurses, something we can truly be grateful for in a modern society.

The correct answer is to rely on both: if you had a serious physical illness, you would do two things, wouldn't you? You'd pray. And you'd go see a doctor. It's just the same with mental health: talk to a medical professional (to the extent that you need to - you know your own symptoms, I don't), and talk also to God about it in prayer.

"Keep me as the apple of your eye; hide me in the shadow of your wings" - *Psalm 17:8*

Did you know that you are the apple of God's eye? Well, hopefully now you do! God loves you, always, no matter what.

Chapter 5 -
You're never 'not good enough' for God

"But God chose the foolish things of the world to shame the wise; God chose the weak things of the world to shame the strong." - 1 Corinthians 1:27

You don't need a psychiatrist to tell you that there's a link between low self-esteem and depression. If you don't like yourself, it's far more likely that you'll be depressed. (The psychiatric evidence is a bit less clear the other way round. Depression *probably* also leads to low self-esteem, but that's slightly less certain - see for example the paper 'Understanding the Link Between Low Self-Esteem and Depression' (Orth and Robins, 2013).

Do you sometimes feel like you hate yourself? Is that feeling more than just a vague passing feeling, but something that's part of your psychological makeup? The Bible has a take on this which is very different from the one you'll hear from non-Christians. We'll look at the full context a bit later on, but in 2 Corinthians 12:9 God says to Paul "*My grace is sufficient for you, for my power is made perfect in weakness.*" Paul then says "I will boast all the more gladly about my weaknesses, so that Christ's power may rest on me."

Paul considers himself to be nothing. Is that low self-esteem? Does he hate himself? Well, no. Not really. Because Paul understands that he is made complete by the Holy Spirit. The power of Jesus Christ is the thing that means we are not actually nothing.

The world will tell you that you have a value, that you're beautiful. They're not wrong, but *why are you beautiful*? Is it because of your physical appearance, something that will gradually change over time as you get old? No - otherwise, older people in society would have no value. Believing that you're beautiful based upon nothing is just words. We have a standard to measure against. That's the difference. You know you're beautiful not because your romantic partner says so (although that's nice), not because your family say so (that's nice too) or because your friends want to make you feel good. You know you're beautiful because God is the judge of such things. And if He says you're beautiful then you are. End of story.

The world will try to con you into believing a lie, that your beauty is based upon other physical things which will also change over time. They'll want to sell you all kinds of makeup and cosmetics, which are designed to cover up any physical blemishes and imperfections. You're beautiful, according to the world, but only if you cover up your physical features with expensive products. It's not true beauty. It's consumer-beauty, beauty that comes at a price. They're not selling you actual beauty. They're selling a concept, the idea that maybe you can *feel* beautiful if only you put time and energy and money into making you look like something you're not.

Is makeup wrong? No, of course not. The last thing we want is for Christians to be puritanical and judgmental, bringing in more unnecessary rules that we'll find it difficult to follow. Just, you shouldn't believe the lie that makeup is the source of beauty or a foundation (sorry) for a positive self-image. Those little physical imperfections are okay, because it's what's on the inside that matters.

I want to share with you some of the lyrics of a Philippa Hanna song, Raggedy Doll, using a child's (or adult's) love for a doll as a way to show how God feels about us:

I've loved you from the day I brought you home,

I've loved you from the day that you were sewn,

every stitch, every seam of you

is just how I dreamed of you.

And so I want the whole wide world to know

I love you from your head down to your toes;

I love you from your head down to your toes.

'Cause you are beautifully and wonderfully made.

I don't make mistakes and I wouldn't change a thing.

It makes me sadder when I hear you say

you wish you were stitched some other way

'cause you don't look like the other toys

and you're not new any more.

I wanna take you down from the nursery shelf

and show you love 'till you love yourself

and if you lose a button I will give you mine

just because you're mine.

And you are beautifully and wonderfully made.

I don't make mistakes and I wouldn't change a thing.

I wish Philippa Hanna knew just how inspirational that song, and those words, have been to friends of mine who battle with issues of self-esteem. That reminds me how lonely writing (or preaching or singing or anything where you pour the contents of your heart out to a group of people you might not know) can be sometimes. At the start of the Covid-19 pandemic I rushed out a book '40 days in the desert' as a devotional to help people through lockdown. It was imperfect. That's what happens when you produce an entire book in 72 hours. Though ironically, the big mistake wasn't in the writing. When exporting the file for print, I 'lost' one of the days and accidentally printed the same page twice whilst missing out another one. Most people didn't notice, or were too polite to point out that they'd noticed.

These things happen when you're in a rush. Once I realised the mistake, it set me off into a spiral of days of depression. I felt bad about what had happened. It was unprofessional, and there for everyone to see. That's even worse (to me) than a physical imperfection. It was my error, and I couldn't blame anyone else.

That book had lots of imperfections. So does this book. Every book does. You might not like my writing style. The short sentences. The conversational approach. The use of punctuation. You might find a typo that I've missed because my design software doesn't have a spellcheck. I didn't really know how much impact that book had made.

Then, just as I was trying to work out whether God wants me to write this book or not, two years on, I had a message passed on to me from someone who I hadn't seen or spoken to for twenty years, telling me how that book had been confirmation from God about a major life-changing decision. That seemed like God's timing. God works like that: confirmation through coincidence.

Does God really want me to write this book? Well, there are only two possibilities. Either, yes, in which case I'd better obey Him. Or no, in which case it's just a human idea of mine which hopefully will still be able to bless those who read it. So I'm taking the risk, writing these words, and when we take risks...that's when we're truly vulnerable. Because we start thinking: *What if...?*

What if people don't like this book?

What if I make a mistake in the theology?

What if something I say accidentally upsets someone?

What if it's just a waste of time and money and doesn't achieve its actual aim?

Every 'what if' plays back in to low self-esteem. It's paralysing, causing us to not start projects (or not finish them). It causes us to worry once we've done our part and it's left to other people.

In the Bible, when God clearly told people in an audible voice 'Do This', they knew that the 'what ifs' were just lack of faith. When God told Joshua to march around the walled city of Jericho a total of 13 times, with some trumpet blowing at the end, it must have seemed like madness. There would have been plenty of 'what ifs', but Joshua obeyed because it was clear that God had told him what to do.

Now what about our 'what ifs'? Ours are the situations where we have a level of uncertainty: we might feel that God is telling us to do something, but we might be unsure. We can test those things (and should): Is this in accordance with the Bible? Does it fit with the character of God? Will this strengthen people? Am I doing this for the right reasons? How do I feel when I pray about this? Do other Christians share my vision? All of those answers will help, but sometimes we still aren't absolutely sure. We risk embarrassment.

Then there are the doubts. Am I capable of doing this thing? Can I really step out in faith or will the hurdles be a step too far to overcome? That kind of doubt is rarely of God. We know that, in ourselves, we are nothing. That's already factored in: even the Apostle Paul said that He chose the foolish things of this world to shame the wise, and that He chose the weak to shame the strong (1 Corinthians 1:27, quoted in the title page of this chapter). Every doubt about our own ability and capacity is not a doubt from God.

I'd offer one very general piece of advice. The Great Commission in Matthew 28 can almost be summed up in just one word: "Go". If the Good News of Jesus Christ is life-changing and transformative, then of course we should share that with all those around us. Go. I'll quote a couple of verses, just because context is important, but the command to 'Go' tells us that we should err on the side of taking that step of faith (no matter how difficult it might seem at the time). It also comes with a promise: as we go, we know that God will be with us. *"Therefore go and make disciples of all nations, baptising them in the name of the Father and of the Son and of the Holy Spirit, and teaching them to obey everything I have commanded you. And surely I am with you always, to the very end of the age." - Matthew 28:19-20*

When we're suffering from low self-esteem, it's like we're only seeing one half of the sentence. I am nothing, but in Christ I am everything. The way we see the first half of that sentence changes completely with the second half. How, then, could you possibly be not good enough for Him? He asks of you one thing: Go.

Now I don't know what 'Go' means for you. Honestly, I'm not even sure half the time what 'Go' means for me either. Sometimes, in terms of a spiritual calling and long-term approach, that matters a lot. But in a general, day-to-day sense, 'Go' might simply mean being there for a friend who needs you. 'Go' can mean many little things throughout the day. 'Go' makes us vulnerable, but when we 'Go' that's when we become fulfilled. We go to church, we receive something of God, and then what happens next? Receiving and giving are two sides of the same coin.

Chapter 6 - Father God

"Will God really fulfil his promises to take care of me-- to protect me under all conditions?" Madame Bilquis Sheikh, in 'I dared to call Him Father'

Converting from Islam to Christianity is not the safest thing to do in Pakistan. At the time, media attention was focused on the case of Asia Bibi, who had been sentenced to death for allegedly violating Pakistan's 'blasphemy' laws. She was not the only one to face persecution: even today, in 2022, Pakistan is ranked as the 8th-worst country in the world when it comes to persecuting Christians, according to the Open Doors charity.

So when Bilquis Sheikh found that the God she was looking for could not be found in the pages of the Koran but in the Bible, she risked everything by converting to Christianity. She dared to call God her father, as the title of her book shows. In such circumstances, trusting in God's protection is a whole different world from what we know in Western society. There are times in history when Christians have been called upon to make the ultimate sacrifice, to die for their faith. I'm reminded of Cassie Bernall, who was staring down the barrel of a school shooter's gun in America and challenged whether she believed in God. She said yes, and was murdered. I'm thinking of the Apostle Paul, who 'could have been set free' if he had not appealed to Caesar (Acts 26:32) but instead was sent to Rome. We don't know for sure the details, because they aren't recorded in the Bible, but it seems that Paul was executed in Rome, possibly beheaded on the authority of Nero. I don't know what Paul said or did whilst in Rome, but quite likely it was pivotal to the spread of Christianity over the next two thousand years. Yet those, like Paul, who were killed because of their faith will receive their reward in heaven. Remember, 'forever' is more important than 'right now'.

Apart from those occasional examples, where martyrdom was specifically part of God's plan, we know that we enjoy God's protection. God protected Bilquis Sheikh. God protected prophets, time and again through the Old Testament. God protected Paul many times earlier in his ministry. And even in the rainbow, the symbol of God's promise to humanity, we see God's protection. Why wouldn't God protect us? He is, after all, Our Father. When Jesus teaches us how to pray, He tells us to begin with those words. God is not some distant figure sitting on an isolated throne in the crowds, however much He might be portrayed that way in the media. We can approach God as our father.

Matthew 7:11 tells us what this means for us. *"If you, then, though you are evil, know how to give good gifts to your children, how much more will your Father in heaven give good gifts to those who ask him!"*

That parent-child relationship between God and ourselves is the reason that we can approach Him directly. We don't need (and whilst I respect Catholics, they miss the point when it comes to priests taking 'confession' to provide a link between God and us) anyone else. 1 Timothy 2:5 tells us that no, we can approach God directly:

"For there is one God and one mediator between God and mankind, the man Christ Jesus". In Hebrews 4:16 we're told to *"approach God's throne of grace with confidence, so that we may receive mercy and find grace to help us in our time of need"*.

In his book *The Father Heart of God*, Floyd McClung points out something that I'd never really thought of before. When we say that God is our father, that should have a positive meaning. It should be a loving relationship. And yet one of the root causes of depression *can* often be a dysfunctional family life growing up. Not in my case, I hasten to add, but that can be the case. Those who have never had a father or mother as a positive role model might actually struggle to understand what such love should actually look like.

Floyd McClung talks of those whose parents died when they were young, of people who had been abused by the very people supposed to protect them, or people growing up simply in a loveless family where they felt unwanted. People growing up in those situations might simply have no concept of what the 'father' means in 'father God'.

You may have heard the phrase 'Abba Father', where in many churches the word 'Abba' is described as being like 'daddy'. There are problems with that translation, because 'Abba' is also a word which would have been used by adults in a polite form of address. But it does also indicate the closeness of that bond between Father God and us, His children. There is a full spectrum of roles played by the father. Does He give us good gifts? Absolutely. Does he love us, care for us and want to protect us? Yes. But it also means that there are times when He will set boundaries for us, just like if you are a loving parent you would keep your child away from running across the road because you know that ultimately it would be unsafe to do so.

Can you relate to the concept of a loving father? If so, that's great. If not, then maybe it's important to try to understand what God as our Father means in every aspect of fatherhood.

- Yes, there is an element of 'daddy' looking after a young child
- He's the proud father watching from the touchline, our greatest cheerleader, shouting encouragement as we play for our team
- Our father sets rules and boundaries for us, not in some authoritarian way but because following those rules keeps us safe
- When we were children, we knew little. God as a father is a source of wisdom, support and advice
- He teaches us the things we need to know in order to become grown-up, mature in our faith

Chapter 7 - The problem of suffering

"I consider that our present sufferings are not worth comparing with the glory that will be revealed in us." - Romans 8:18

My grandad was an atheist, or so he said. None of us believed him. The way he spoke wasn't the way that an atheist would talk. He'd lived through the Second World War, fought in every major engagement from the Normandy landings, and seen countless colleagues and friends die. The war wasn't senseless. It was a war against one of the greatest evils the world had ever seen. But victory had its price: all the soldiers who came home in body bags, leaving widows and orphans behind. The civilians killed by the dreadful bombings of British cities. The terrible calculations of the use of nuclear weapons in Hiroshima and Nagasaki to save the lives of countless more who would have died had the fighting continued to the bitter end.

Then there was the cost to those who survived. Those who had been prisoners of war, those who lived for six years not knowing whether they would ever see their fathers, sons or husbands again, and those who had survived the concentration camps. They would never forget, and the psychological scars would run deep. My grandad would, I'm sure, have been diagnosed with post-traumatic stress disorder in today's society. After every piece of death and inhumanity that he had seen, month after month, year after year, something inside him would never be the same again. He would sleepwalk, wandering into the middle of the street, or wake up screaming. War is a certain kind of hell on earth, and he had lived through it. Even fifty years later, we could still see for ourselves the toll that it had taken on him.

He was sad. He was also angry. He was angry at God for allowing all that suffering to happen. He was so angry at God that he started to deny God's existence, loudly. Every so often, his guard would slip - just a touch - and that anger would seep through rather than the denial. He had once had a faith in God, and now he turned away because of the horrible things he had seen.

I like to think that, in the time sixty years after that horrific war, when my grandad lay dying in his hospital bed, that he made his peace with God. We certainly had a sense of peace about the situation, but nobody knows for sure what is in someone else's heart. My grandad had experienced first-hand the question which theologians and philosophers have debated since the very beginning of Christianity: if God exists, and if God is good, why does He permit such suffering to take place in this world? Why doesn't He intervene to stop all these awful things happening?

Why, you might ask when going through a particularly rough phase and suffering with your mental health, does God allow me to go through all of this? There are answers, but they aren't easy answers.

It all goes back to the Garden of Eden, to the fall of humanity. Adam and Eve didn't obey God. They brought sin into the world. They introduced the concept that humans might choose to ignore God's way and decide to do things our own way instead. God could have overruled them, like someone playing the Sims computer game can 'force' those Sims to change their tasks. Then yes, Adam and Eve would have been perfect: they would have done precisely God's will, because they would have had no choice but to do God's will.

They would, like the Sims, have been nothing more than robots: some computerised construction with no actual meaning whatsoever. That's not a relationship between God and us. It's just basically a computer programme. So God made the other choice. a choice which we might think of as heartbreaking. He allowed us to make our own decisions, even when that meant we might choose sometimes to turn our backs on Him.

That decision led to suffering. It led to joy. It led to a real, meaningful relationship between God and us. And it led to suffering: the blot on the landscape - sin - meant our imperfect choices would hurt others. Sin would have consequences, and sometimes those consequences would have an impact on other situations. We, as human beings, made that choice to step away from God's protection and into our own world instead. The gap between God and us was so huge that He sent His only son, Jesus Christ, to experience a level of suffering which went beyond anything else we've talked about in this book. To be *"pierced for our transgressions, crushed for our iniquities*", as Isaiah prophesied (Isaiah 53:5). And from that agonising death which Jesus suffered on the cross, we know one encouraging thing: that however bad our suffering might get, God understands: Jesus went through far worse when He gave His life so that we might live - not just here on this earth, but forever.

It's that word 'forever' which matters. When you see a doctor, you might experience some short-term pain but with a long-term health benefit. A moment of suffering is worth years of a healthier life. In the same way, even if you suffer during years on earth, we can know that as believers our reward in heaven will make that suffering seem so tiny and insignificant in comparison that it will barely even register. Have you ever heard this joke?

I was standing in the park, wondering why a frisbee seems to get bigger, the closer to you it gets? And then...it hit me.

There's a word for that: perspective. When something is right in front of you, it feels bigger than when it's far away. If we could see through God's eyes, having 'forever' in mind, we would be able to understand how amazing our reward is in heaven - and how little the suffering actually matters.

And that helps. Sort of. I mean, it helps on an intellectual level. You might believe that in your head, but when you're suffering - whether that's physical pain or mental anguish - it doesn't *feel* like that. Does how you feel right this minute make a difference to the eternal plan? No, but it's pretty important to you right this second. There's a gap between *knowing* that God is good, and being able to *feel* His loving arms around you.

If you aren't a parent, imagine that you're a mother of a small child. Sometimes that child will want things that you can't provide. Maybe you know that something would be unhealthy or dangerous and you want nothing more than to protect the son or daughter who you love from something bad happening to them. Maybe your child is screaming the place down because he or she doesn't want to go to school, or maybe that same child 'wants' something like an ice-cream or a new toy. Sometimes those things are okay, but other times they aren't. And in those moments, the child might - in a fit of anger - start to think that you don't really love them. How many times throughout history have children and teenagers yelled "I hate you" at parents? They are loved. Always. As a parent you're going to love your child no matter what, even when they make bad choices.

Here's the kicker though. The child won't always *feel* loved. Feelings are a really bad indicator. Sometimes you might feel loved by someone who doesn't truly care, just because they spoke the right word at the right time. Other times, you might feel distant from your husband or wife, with one of you angry about some insignificant nonsense and the other stressed out through being overworked. It doesn't make you any less loved, but at times like those the feeling isn't there. The difference with God is, I suppose, that it's one-sided. You might be irrational towards your partner, or your partner might be irrational towards you, and that's part and parcel of a marriage (or a relationship heading in that direction). It happens. Both of you will make mistakes. Whether it's 50-50 or 90-10, nobody is capable of perfection. Nobody except God Himself. But isn't it possible that, in the same way, things in our real lives make 'feelings' a bad way of understanding just how much God loves us? Sometimes we might feel it. Sometimes we might not. But nothing will ever change the fact that God loves us so much:

"For I am convinced that neither death nor life, neither angels nor demons, neither the present nor the future, nor any powers, neither height nor depth, nor anything else in all creation, will be able to separate us from the love of God that is in Christ Jesus our Lord." - Romans 8:38-39

The Apostle Paul is certainly sure about that: nothing whatsoever can separate us from God's love. And that is 100% true, whether you feel it right now or not. Some people believe that Paul himself suffered from depression. I don't like assuming things that go beyond what's written in the Bible (remember that warning in Revelation not to add or take away from what's in it?), but certainly Paul faced many tough situations - some of which left him feeling despair, even though he remained faithful to God. Look at 2 Corinthians 1:8-9, which says:

We were under great pressure, far beyond our ability to endure, so that we despaired of life itself. Indeed, we felt we had received the sentence of death. But this happened that we might not rely on ourselves but on God, who raises the dead.

Paul 'despaired of life itself'. And yet, what did that do? Did it make him turn away from God? No, he learned to rely *even more* on God. A difficult thing for us to copy, especially when we're depressed, but it will help. The other verse sometimes quoted is the 'thorn in the flesh'. The meaning of this passage has been debated for centuries. Does it mean a real person? Does it mean an evil spirit? Does it mean a physical affliction? Does it mean a sin that Paul was tempted constantly to commit? Does it mean suffering from depression? I don't think we can know for sure, but judge for yourself from the passage:

"Therefore, in order to keep me from becoming conceited, I was given a thorn in my flesh, a messenger of Satan, to torment me. Three times I pleaded with the Lord to take it away from me. But he said to me, "My grace is sufficient for you, for my power is made perfect in weakness." Therefore I will boast all the more gladly about my weaknesses, so that Christ's power may rest on me. That is why, for Christ's sake, I delight in weaknesses, in insults, in hardships, in persecutions, in difficulties. For when I am weak, then I am strong." - 2 Corinthians 12:7-10

If I'm honest, I think that passage *probably* isn't referring to depression but it is still a brilliant description of how I feel when I'm depressed. Depression might torment me, and I might plead with God to take that away, and yet the answer would still be that God's grace is enough. God *could* cure every single symptom of depression right now, and I guess that's what we want him to do. Deep down, we're desperate for that to happen. It doesn't, at least not as regularly as we'd like. The Bible doesn't promise that every single time something is wrong, God will cure it like waving some hypothetical 'magic wand'. We shouldn't reduce God to some kind of wish-granting machine; that's not who God is!

"Praise be to the God and Father of our Lord Jesus Christ, the Father of compassion and the God of all comfort, who comforts us in all our troubles, so that we can comfort those in any trouble with the comfort we ourselves receive from God. For just as we share abundantly in the sufferings of Christ, so also our comfort abounds through Christ." - 2 Corinthians 1:3-5

Yes. That's it. God doesn't take our troubles away, or at least not all the time. Paul, who wrote those words, was flogged, imprisoned, beaten, shipwrecked, hungry and many other things before (according to external sources to the Bible) eventually being executed in Rome for being a Christian. God certainly didn't take all Paul's troubles away. But He did provide the comfort which Paul needed. God doesn't take away our suffering, In fact, we share in Christ's suffering.

Why? Now this is the part which I really hope will motivate you. Why does God comfort us through all our troubles? Is it because God loves us? Well yes, but that's not the reason that Paul gives. Paul gives a reason that looks outwards, beyond ourselves, to the others out there who need a touch from God as well. God comforts us *so that we can comfort others* who are also in trouble.

That's it. That's your mission. If you're suffering, it is also part of your 'job' as a Christian to comfort others who are going through the same kind of thing. I feel that this is the main reason why we're allowed to go through all of this. Remember back at the very start of this book, when I said that I had to sit down five times to try to write because every other time I'd been interrupted by having to care for and comfort different friends who were suffering with something related to depression? If ever there was confirmation that I should be writing this book, that was it! I think, though, that although it's not 'God's divine will' that I should suffer from depression (that would be a pretty cruel thing), it's 'God's permissive will' (He allows me to go through that, knowing that it will provide me with the ability to comfort others).

There may be much more to it than that, but at the heart there are three things you should remember:

- God knows exactly what you're going through. He understands you.
- He will comfort you through your depression.
- We can't know all the reasons we suffer from depression, but we do know that through it we can help to comfort others.

Chapter 8 -
In the world but not of it

"If you belonged to the world, it would love you as its own. As it is, you do not belong to the world, but I have chosen you out of the world. That is why the world hates you." - John 15:19

I'm sure you'll have heard that phrase. The one where Christians are called to be 'in the world, but not of it'. It isn't actually a Bible verse. There are plenty of Bible verses which say the same thing (and more), so it's perfectly reasonable. I think the verse in John 15 suggests something even more than that. It says that God has *chosen* us out of the world. It's not an accident. It's not a situation where we just happen to be sharing the same planet as non-Christians. No, God has chosen us.

1 Peter 2:9 tells us that we are "*a chosen people, a royal priesthood, a holy nation, God's special possession*". You are God's special possession. In those times when you feel worthless, when you feel like you can't understand how anyone could possibly want you, the creator of the universe describes you as being chosen, royal, holy - and His special possession. How amazing!

If we could read those words, understand them and truly take them to heart, there would be no need for this book. The problem is that in this 'fallen world' ('fallen' refers to Adam and Eve, with a perfect world becoming an imperfect one), it's sometimes difficult for us to truly believe that we are that: precious and special to God. That gap between what we know in our heads, and what we feel in our hearts, is in essence the spiritual cause of depression.

Every day though, we live in a world that we don't quite fit in with. We don't value the same things that this world values. Are we searching to make as much money as we possibly can? No. We're trying to store up 'treasures in heaven' (Matthew 6:19-21) which can never be stolen from us. What does that mean? Well, it means that the world will never understand us. If you're struggling with depression, it's quite likely that you feel that people don't 'understand' you. And it's true that non-Christians won't really understand what makes Christians 'tick'. How could they? How could someone who has never known Jesus, never had the Holy Spirit within them, understand how we perceive the word? They can't. Maybe that plays into those feelings of being out-of-step with the world. That's where your 'church family' can come in, provided that they're sensitive to what's actually going on. I was talking recently to someone who was going through a particularly rough time, with anxiety and depression. I can't remember the exact words, but it was something like this: "When I'm with other Christians, I feel like it's okay that people know I'm finding things difficult. Even if I've never met them before, they're like my family in God".

Amazing stuff! Of course, being around other Christians can help. We are supposed to have fellowship with each other: to spend time in the company of other believers, whether that's praying, reading the Bible, in worship to God, or just spending time together over a meal. Those relationships between believers are building-blocks. Without them, how can we strengthen and encourage each other? How else can we build each other up before we go back out into a world that can never really understand us? Proverbs 27: 17 says *"As iron sharpens iron, so one person sharpens another".* By working together, we become more than just the sum of our parts. Every church will tell you that 'church is about much more than just the Sunday service', and that's absolutely true. It's also about much more than just the people who happen to attend the same church as you. I spend time in fellowship, in different ways, with friends who go to various churches all around the country. Sometimes that's more in a mentoring-type way, in the sense that Paul helped Timothy to grow in his faith. Sometimes the dynamic is two people working together to face the world, in the same way as Paul and Silas. Sometimes it's just friendship within the framework of God. That fellowship can take different forms. When it's within 'your' church, that's a blessing because it becomes something that's in the culture and life of the congregation - but it doesn't have to be exclusively within that church either.

Fellowship is so important in breaking through depression. It's important also as a reset, because living within the world is particularly difficult. Years ago, when I was involved in politics (and that can be a good thing for Christians to do), I found that it weighed heavily on me. There was a constant pressure to be nasty towards people with a different colour rosette, or towards someone who just happened to have a different opinion. There was one moral dilemma after another, and it was a constant challenge to make sure to act in a Godly way. Did I get it right every single time? No, of course not...but I can only hope that those who were with me on that particular journey were able to see something 'different' about me because I am a Christian. John 13:34-35 says *"A new command I give you: Love one another. As I have loved you, so you must love one another. By this everyone will know that you are my disciples, if you love one another"*. That means resisting the constant pressure to act in an un-Christian, unloving manner. It also means standing up for what is right, defending those who can't defend themselves, even when it comes at a personal cost to do so.

Politics was an extreme example of it, but we all face the weight of a world that wants and expects us to conform to the standards of the world. Fighting against that, choosing to follow God's path instead, is absolutely 100% the right thing to do. It's also exhausting.

I was chatting to a good Christian friend who was going through a mental health crisis. I'd spent most of the evening trying to help her through a time of self-harm, and over a period of a few hours we'd got to a stage of being able to pray and things started to seem better. But then, in the early hours of the morning, she received an abusive message from a non-Christian. He had been offended by her faith: how could she post about people being 'saved' when there's so much suffering in the world? The language was more angry, and contained threats to basically stalk her online. I get that the question of suffering is a difficult one, for all of us, as we already discussed in an earlier chapter. But instead, he wanted to persecute my friend for being a Christian. He wanted, ironically, to create suffering for her (whilst arguing that he was a 'good' person because he thought he was opposed to suffering). That sort of twisted logic really doesn't help anyone, but it's a great example of the difference between what a Christian does and what 'the world' does.

That level of persecution is nothing to what you might see in North Korea or any of dozens of nations worldwide where Christians face a very real threat of imprisonment or death for simply believing in Jesus. In the Sermon on the Mount, Jesus deals with it directly (Matthew 5:10-11):

"Blessed are those who are persecuted because of righteousness, for theirs is the kingdom of heaven. Blessed are you when people insult you, persecute you and falsely say all kinds of evil against you because of me."

That's absolutely right. When you go through those times and stand firm in your faith, you are richly blessed. It just...well, it doesn't feel like it sometimes when it's 3 o'clock in the morning and you still can't get to sleep. Feelings, though, are very different from reality. You are blessed in those situations, and God will give you what you need to get through. In fact, when you are being persecuted for your faith, you should know that it's evidence you're actually doing something right. 1 Peter 3:17 tells us that it *"is better, if it is God's will, to suffer for doing good than for doing evil"*. In 1 Peter 4, he expands on that point (verses 12-16):

"Dear friends, do not be surprised at the fiery ordeal that has come on you to test you, as though something strange were happening to you. But rejoice inasmuch as you participate in the sufferings of Christ, so that you may be overjoyed when his glory is revealed. If you are insulted because of the name of Christ, you are blessed, for the Spirit of glory and of God rests on you. If you suffer, it should not be as a murderer or thief or any other kind of criminal, or even as a meddler. However, if you suffer as a Christian, do not be ashamed, but praise God that you bear that name."

If you, for example, had been caught stealing then you'd get into trouble with the law for doing it. The consequence of that action would probably be unpleasant: you might go to court and end up with a criminal record. That's a natural result that occurs when you commit a crime. Where's the blessing in that? There is none. But if you're in trouble because you stood up for your faith in God, then you would be blessed! It's not something that we should be surprised about: the world doesn't understand, and when the world doesn't understand it can get nasty. That decision to 'turn the other cheek' is always a difficult one. But Peter goes one step further: you don't need to be ashamed at that persecution. In fact, you can praise God! Even through a 'fiery ordeal', as Peter describes it, you have stood firm. Even those who aren't believers can see that - and respect it. Some of the jailers who beat and tortured the Romanian pastor Richard Wurmbrand in Soviet times were so amazed by him that they became Christians themselves.

Then there is the other problem, the problem that the Government and the Church don't always see eye-to-eye. Sometimes that's easy enough for us to resolve. There are plenty of things which *the Bible tells us are sinful*, but which also are *not illegal*, and that's actually okay. If we aren't supposed to do something, that is between us and God. The law doesn't need to get involved.

Suppose that someone you know, a Christian, is having a string of affairs. Should they be carted off to prison for it? No, of course not. Should the Church be having some serious words with that person? Well, yes. There's a sense of spiritual accountability. That's straightforward stuff. We are in the world but not of it, and we need to hold ourselves to a higher standard.

Now what if it's a non-Christian having an affair? Trickier, isn't it? The Bible offers us a moral standard: someone who as a Christian engages in sexual intercourse other than in a marriage relationship (and there is plenty of discussion about what is and isn't okay pre-marriage even in Christianity) is sinning. But how do we know it's wrong? We only know it's wrong because the Bible tells us so. Marriage only means anything because it's the institution that God established in the first place - it's literally part of the wedding vows in most churches. If someone is living outside God's law, it's not our place to blame them for not following God's law.

The problem is, that when we don't follow God's law, consequences arise. That non-Christian might risk a messy marriage break-up, or catching an STD, or any of a number of things that could happen as a consequence of stepping away from God's general protection. It's only immoral, though, when viewed through the lens of Christianity. Even if it hurts someone, why is hurting someone wrong? What is the standard? How do we know that hurting someone else is a bad thing to do, unless it comes back to God's directions for us? It might 'feel' bad, or it might be something that society tells us is bad, but who is the referee if it's not God? That brings us back to the problem: if your non-Christian friend is doing something 'sinful', there's a real tightrope to walk. You don't want to be judgmental, but you also know that there is a better way to live your life.

Then what about situations where the world very deliberately sets its own 'moral' standards in contradiction to the Bible? Right from the very first book of the Bible (Genesis 1:27) - "male and female, he created them". We know that the world is no longer perfect, and that imperfection can be seen scientifically through all kinds of genetic problems which have crept into our DNA. So we also know that a tiny proportion of people are born 'intersex', having both male and female characteristics, and sometimes doctors might make the wrong decision in guessing male or female at birth.

Then, there are people who - although born as male - feel like they're female, or vice versa. Again, it's more difficult for a Christian to respond. Is that part and parcel of the 'fallen world', that a mistake has crept in somewhere along the line, or is it part of a world which has different standards to God's law? We can reconcile those views, I think.

But then society takes it one step further. We're told to accept the existence of various other genders (72, I think), and now that presents us with a problem as Christians. Society expects us to ignore the Bible, to ignore everything that speaks of male and female. Concepts such as the church being the 'bride of Christ' (2 Corinthians 11:2, Ephesians 5:27, Revelation 19:7, etc.) which are reinforced in the Bible would become meaningless if we threw away the Bible's teaching. Now society is on a directly contradictory path with Christianity. But what do I do, when one of my friends decides that she now identifies as 'genderfluid' or wants to be addressed using different pronouns? It leaves me with a huge dilemma. On the one hand, I should stand up for my faith and I should not accept my beliefs being watered down by 'the world'. We are Christians. We aren't of 'the world'. We are set apart from it. On the other hand, I'm supposed to 'love my neighbour as myself'. I should show love towards my fellow human beings. What a terrible witness it would be, if I were to respond with anger or mocking at a friend who is clearly struggling through a particular situation! I would be no better than the person who messaged my friend earlier in the chapter, persecuting her for her faith in Christianity. Because we live in an imperfect world, these problems can weigh heavily on our minds. I don't have a perfect answer, but I try to work out how to act. I try to treat people with respect and dignity, but to do so in a way that does not go against their beliefs.

Depending on your generation, this might be an issue you come across on a regular basis or it might not. I've come across this issue four times in the last six months in my personal life: each time, it's presented me with a spiritual dilemma. [I've known transgender people for many years, and that doesn't cause the same direct challenge to Christianity: it isn't denying the nature of 'male' and 'female', but someone born as 'male' saying that they believe they are 'female'- or vice versa.]

Same problem, different context: suppose a non-Christian friend tells you that she's going to have an abortion. When Psalm 139 tells us about how God 'knits us together' in our mother's womb and how God weaves us together, it's natural to conclude that abortion goes against God's plan. But how do you talk to that friend, especially if she's finding things difficult, knowing that she's living to a different moral standard? There are things you maybe can do, such as offer practical help with looking after the baby. Even so, as a Christian your world-view is going to come into conflict with your friend's world-view. You might well choose to minimise that conflict as part of showing God's love, and that's where showing positive, loving, practical support comes in. In those situations, everything is walking a tightrope and there is no easy answer. The problem is that, as Christians, we don't have the option of simply sitting back and saying nothing. Even if you were just thinking about a friend and not her baby, do you really want her to suffer the psychological trauma that is so common in mothers who have had an abortion? God gives us all free will. We can make our own choices. We're not robots, but if someone was about to walk into the path of an oncoming car you'd certainly warn them of the danger. The difference is that people understand the dangers of being run over by a car, but they might not recognise when the hurt will be psychological or spiritual rather than physical. There is no simple formula for how we show God's love in those circumstances. If you push something too hard, you risk losing a friend and being unable to care for her later in her time of need.

Such situations are heartbreaking, and I could give many similar examples of where the world's view conflicts with God's view. When that happens, it is difficult and working out how to 'be a good friend' in those situations can be a trigger for depression.

We can:

- Be encouraged: you are chosen, holy and "God's special possession". You matter so much to Him.

- Spend time with other Christians, in fellowship with them, building each other up.

- Remember that whenever bad things happen because we're Christians, we are blessed by God.

- Try to live our lives according to His plan, but without causing unnecessary offence to non-believers around us.

- Understand that we can't hold non-Christians to God's standards, and try to gently guide people away from danger.

Chapter 9 - Guilt and forgiveness

"But where sin increased, grace increased all the more, so that, just as sin reigned in death, so also grace might reign through righteousness to bring eternal life through Jesus Christ our Lord." - Romans 5:20-21

It's natural for human beings to feel guilty. We have a lot to feel guilty about. If we're brutally honest, how many of us has gone a full day without sinning? When we remember that sinful thoughts are still sin, it's pretty difficult to go even a single hour without sinning. That's who we are, and when those sins don't affect other people, it's easy not to feel guilty about them. Many of them are sins of omission (I really can't be bothered to...) where you don't do things that you really should. Sin happens, yes because we live in a fallen world, but also because the standard we fail to reach is perfection. And, as people will never tire of telling you, nobody's perfect. That's only half the story: we are imperfect, but through God it's like those sins never existed when we repent of them:

"I, even I, am he who blots out your transgressions, for my own sake, and remembers your sins no more." - Isaiah 43:25

"For by one sacrifice he has made perfect forever those who are being made holy." - Hebrews 10:14

I have swept away your offenses like a cloud, your sins like the morning mist. Return to me, for I have redeemed you." - Isaiah 44:22

They're gone. So why do we still feel guilty? First of all, it's important to understand that there are (at least) three different kinds of guilt:

1. When we feel 'guilty' because our actions weren't right, and because we feel that we let ourselves or God down.

2. When we feel 'guilty' because our actions had a negative impact on people around us, and we see that we caused hurt to another person.

3. When we feel 'guilty' over a situation that we could never have controlled, but we were involved with. (Think of a situation where you go out for the afternoon, then come back to find that someone you live with has fallen over and broken a bone: you might feel 'guilty' that you weren't there, because

you could have helped, but it wasn't your 'fault' because there was no way of knowing that was going to happen.

I don't think guilt is absolutely 100% unhealthy 100% of the time. It's usually unhealthy, but there are exceptional times (I believe) when God does allow us to feel guilty about a situation which we've caused if it helps us to learn and grow, to avoid doing the same thing again. The Bible uses the word 'discipline', which is often talked about but very rarely defined in this context:

"If you are not disciplined—and everyone undergoes discipline—then you are not legitimate, not true sons and daughters at all...no discipline seems pleasant at the time, but painful. Later on, however, it produces a harvest of righteousness and peace for those who have been trained by it." - Hebrews 12:8 and 11

It's just the nature of having a loving God as our father that He will gently steer us away from the things we shouldn't do, towards the things that we should. The most 'famous' Psalm of all, Psalm 23, describes the Lord as being 'our shepherd'. A shepherd looks after and cares for all the sheep in the flock, guiding them away from danger and into safe pastures where they can live and graze.

Don't think of a shepherd in Biblical times as being the same as modern farming. It was much more hands-on. The sheep needed to be protected from danger, so a shepherd would be armed with a 'rod'. If you remember the Flintstones, imagine Fred Flintstone's club. Something heavy (often with nails in it) would be useful to ward off any predators who fancied raw lamb for dinner. The shepherd might also be armed with a sling, like David used to defeat Goliath. He would often sleep in the fields with his sheep, keeping them safe overnight. It was a very active, daily form of protection.

When God speaks about being our shepherd, it means more than you'd think the first time you read those words. There's a loving relationship between shepherd and sheep in the Bible (think of the Parable of the Lost Sheep, in which the farmer can find only 99 of the 100 sheep and goes out to search for the one that is missing, because each and every sheep is precious to him). But there's also a sense in which the farmer is robust, insisting that his sheep do not run away. The sheep might love the idea of gambolling with their lives (sorry, again!) by leaving the shepherd's protection and roaming free through the countryside. Unfortunately they would be caught and eaten by lions or other predators. The shepherd would use a staff to guide, firmly but as gently as possible, his sheep back into the fold. The staff was what you might imagine today as a walking stick: a long stick with a curved handle.

The Bible invites us to think of God's care for us (and discipline of us) like a good shepherd who always has his flock in mind. In practical terms, if we have genuinely done something hurtful to another person, God would of course forgive our sins completely - whilst at the same time, there is a natural consequence that our behaviour has caused something bad to happen. We have the responsibility not to just seek God's forgiveness, but also to put things right with the other person and seek restoration or reconciliation. During that process, we might well feel guilty about our actions and that could be part and parcel of the process of growing and learning. The Bible talks about a refiner's fire, burning away all the impurities in silver to make sure that the finished product is ideal. When we are 'going through the fire', to use the modern phrase, it might not be pleasant but it moulds us into being better human beings. That's why I say guilt isn't absolutely a bad thing 100% of the time, because it can (in some situations) actually be useful.

The other kinds of guilt are clearly bad though, again in my opinion. It's very important to 'test' what anyone tells you, whether that's a preacher or the author of a book. In some situations, where I'm offering a personal interpretation, I'd rather flag that up so that you can test what I'm saying for yourself (see: 1 Thessalonians 5:18-21 for more on testing).

Suppose you feel guilty simply because you sinned. Nobody else has been hurt in the process. What do you do? You seek God's forgiveness. And God forgives you because it is the nature of God to forgive. That's grace: the more we sin, the more there is to be forgiven. We can never exhaust God's forgiveness: however much sin increases, so does His grace (Romans 5:20-21). There's a situation where we find ourselves committing the same type of sin, over and over again. Perhaps it's more convenient to lie than admit the truth. Perhaps it's a struggle with sexual sin. Or jealousy. Or any of dozens of things which even Christians can find that they do over and over again, as though they were in the film Groundhog Day. I think even Paul found that difficult, as he describes his turmoil in Romans 7:15-22 (though the whole chapter is relevant):

I do not understand what I do. For what I want to do I do not do, but what I hate I do. And if I do what I do not want to do, I agree that the law is good. As it is, it is no longer I myself who do it, but it is sin living in me. For I know that good itself does not dwell in me, that is, in my sinful nature. For I have the desire to do what is good, but I cannot carry it out. For I do not do the good I want to do, but the evil I do not want to do—this I keep on doing. Now if I do what I do not want to do, it is no longer I who do it, but it is sin living in me that does it.

So I find this law at work: Although I want to do good, evil is right there with me. For in my inner being I delight in God's law; but I see another law at work in me, waging war against the law of my mind and making me a prisoner of the law of sin at work within me. What a wretched man I am! Who will rescue me from this body that is subject to death? Thanks be to God, who delivers me through Jesus Christ our Lord!

Just reading those words, I get a sense of Paul's inner struggles with his own sinful nature. Our selfish desires will often conflict with God's law and His plan for us. If you have that kind of internal struggle, don't worry. The Apostle Paul also had it. It doesn't mean that there's anything wrong with you. Actually, it means the opposite: it means that you're self-aware, understanding the huge responsibility that comes with being a Christian. Having said that, as long as we're not abusing God's forgiveness (by saying

'I'm just going to go right ahead and commit this sin because I know I can ask for God's forgiveness later' - easily done), we know that His grace is sufficient for us. Guilt in these circumstances can start to become a bad thing, because there's a danger that guilt leads to feeling badly about yourself. Once you get into a spiral of negativity about yourself, that can trigger low self-esteem. If you suffer from depression, it then pushes you into a point where you're finding that you're depressed. Yet the actual thing that's caused the flare-up of your depression is something which God has already forgiven. And not just forgiven, it's been 'forgotten': as we saw in Isaiah 43:25, a*nd remembers your sins no more*, it's just as though it had never happened. To God, it's all in the past. To us, it's causing feelings of depression.

The situation where something is not actually our fault, but we feel guilty anyway, is pretty much the same thing in practice. If we've sinned, and repented, then we have a clean slate in God. If we haven't sinned, then we have a clean slate in God. It's the same position, but we've arrived at it through different means (for the chessplayer who I know will be reading this book, think of the word *transposition*).

In both situations we know that we are in the clear as far as God is concerned. What happens if you take that 'evidence-based' approach we talked about earlier (the 'take the thought to court' concept in cognitive behavioural therapy) and approach that question from a Christian perspective? Where is the evidence 'against' you? There is none: God has wiped it clean. In that 'thought court', we don't just win the case. There is no case to answer at all! It's important, though also difficult, to do your best to 'train your mind' so that you understand that there's nothing there for you to feel guilty about!

God has forgiven you. That's enough. There is no need to over-rule Him in your mind and 'punish' yourself anyway...

Chapter 10 - Testing times

"Blessed is the man who perseveres under trial, because when he has stood the test, he will receive the crown of life that God has promised to those who love him." - James 1:12

"Why", I was asked by someone who had seen the first few chapters of this book, "have you mentioned Old Testament characters such as Elijah and Jeremiah so much, but not Job?"

In the Old Testament, the entire book of Job is about suffering. Job is described as an outstanding person, one who is moral and blameless, making the right choices and 'shunning' evil. As a human being, he must sin from time to time of course, but his overall character is overwhelmingly good. The devil challenges God: Job is allegedly so blameless only *because* his life is easy. If things were difficult for him, would he still be so good?

In my opinion, Job is a real, historical person. I don't believe that the book of Job is intended to be purely as a story to explain something to us about suffering: he is cross-referenced as an example of faith in Ezekiel 14:14, Ezekiel 14:20 and James 5:11. Would that have happened if Job weren't a real person? I doubt it. If it were intended as a kind of 'morality tale', that wouldn't present a problem: the Bible should always be taken literally when it is speaking literally. It should be taken poetically when speaking poetically, figuratively when speaking figuratively and the New Testament letters should be understood in the context of the people who were originally intended to receive them, as well as in the context that they're books of the Bible. So I believe Job was real, but I wouldn't fall out with another Christian who believes otherwise.

He loses everything: all his riches, his children and his family. Job's friends try to persuade him that he's being punished for some evil that he's done, becoming more of a hindrance than a help. Finally, he loses his health. Everything is going wrong for Job. No wonder, then, that Job feels like there's a disconnect between his righteous actions and bad things that are happening to him. The age-old lament 'why me?', when someone feels victimised because lots of bad things are happening all at once, couldn't apply to anyone more than it does to Job. In one sense, Job's sadness had a clear and specific cause. Is that depression though? Anyone is sad when something really bad happens. If you lose your job or a loved one passes away, there is a natural human feeling of emptiness and sadness. I don't think those things mean you're depressed, in and of themselves. It just means you're going through a tough time. Job's time was even tougher than anything we can reasonably imagine, and I think that's the point of the whole book: *even though* he had a horrific time, he still remained faithful to God. There were times that he felt sorry for himself, times he wished that he could die, but the whole point of the book of Job is about his actions rather than his feelings.

I'd been a little reluctant to use Job as an example, because I'm not totally convinced that the book actually relates to depression: Job's sadness is a very natural human reaction. That's why I hadn't really been planning on mentioning him, even if that sounds a bit odd. But the more I thought about it, the more I realised that it's important to consider those situations when we're going through testing times. Job was being tested, with God always having confidence that he would pass the test. Other times, we go through the 'refiner's fire' which I mentioned before: that difficult times in life can be part of the process of getting out impurities and making us stronger human beings. It's also true, I think, to suggest that we learn how to relate to other people's problems through our own. Remember that verse (Hebrews 4) about how Christ was tempted in every way *just as we are*, and yet was without sin? It gives us some comfort hopefully to know that Jesus went through the things that we're experiencing. Now take that one step further. When you are speaking to one of your non-Christian friends, they might well say 'ah, but you just don't understand. My situation is so bad because...'. They start listing all of their current problems. Maybe that person isn't in a place where they're ready for you to point out that Jesus went through all that. First, perhaps, they need to know that you understand them and what they're going through.

Some things are temporary. You get the flu, you expect to recover - but the two weeks in the meantime aren't exactly going to be fun. One reason that most people aren't emotionally traumatised every time they catch a cold is that they know this isn't a life-long problem. When something is temporary, and you know it's temporary, you can usually look forward to a time when you're feeling better and able to enjoy going back to your favourite restaurant.

That's easy enough for us to do. What if, though, you're struggling with the effects of 'long Covid' and you're not sure when (or if) those symptoms will go away? That's more difficult to process emotionally because there is a worry around it.

If you're preparing to go on holiday, only to find that your flight has been cancelled at the last minute, you'll probably be pretty annoyed. Still, you know that there will be future holidays. You might be angry and vent off some steam by screaming at the nearest available inanimate object, but you know it is only a temporary setback.

Human beings are hard-wired to 'hope' for something to improve. The problem with going through a 'testing time' spiritually is that it can feel like that time will never end. You lose your job, there's something to grieve for. But until you get another one, you can't be *sure* that you will - or that the new job will be as good as the last. However much we need hope, doubt can be crippling.

Now think of the Bible's promises on faith in that context. Think of how they apply to people with depression. Depression has a habit of magnifying doubts and minimising hope. "*Now faith*", Hebrews 11:1 tells us, "*is confidence in what we hope for and assurance about what we do not see*". How can we 'believe' in something we don't yet see? Yet that's exactly what we do when we put our trust in the very existence of God: "*By faith*", we are told in Hebrews 11:3, "*we understand that the universe was formed at God's command, so that what is seen was not made out of what was visible.*"

Interesting, isn't it? Look around you for a moment. I see a fireplace, a sofa, a television, a pair of curtains, a drink and all sorts of things. I see my hand, typing these words on a laptop. I imagine the complexity of the laptop, the detail of my fingerprints. If I had a powerful enough magnifying glass I could zoom in to the atoms and molecules zooming around at high speed. I can't even begin to comprehend just how complicated everything is that I see even around me now, or indeed how complicated my eye is to be able to see everything in front of me. Faith tells me that those things didn't come about by accident. Faith tells me that those things are there because *"In the beginning, God created..."* (Genesis 1:1). That faith, a faith in a powerful creator God who explains everything about the past and present, is (mostly) easy for us as Christians. If we have faith in what God did, so far in the past, isn't it strange how having faith in what God will do today or tomorrow can be so challenging?

Faith can certainly be more than a helping hand during testing times, but let's start with something easier. If having faith in what happened ages ago is easy, but tomorrow is difficult, how about having faith in something a little further down the line? Let's go to the end of the Bible:

"He will wipe every tear from their eyes. There will be no more death or mourning or crying or pain, for the old order of things has passed away." - Revelation 21:4

Can we agree on that? We can manage to have faith about the distant future. Why? Well, partly because we know what it is that we are having faith for. It's clear as a promise of God. What does God promise for you this afternoon? That's more difficult, because we can't turn through the pages of the Bible and find a specific promise that tells us what is going to happen then.

We can find general promises, and there are many of them, throughout the Bible. We can't find a promise that the payroll will work and that we'll get our money on time when we really need it tomorrow. We can't find a promise that the plumber who's due to fix the washing machine will turn up on time. What happens when we're going through testing times is that our minds start to focus on those day-to-day things. They're important, yes, but what's happening is that the details of everyday life move our perspective away from God's. *"Do not worry about your life"*, Matthew 6:25 tells us, *"what you will eat or drink; or about your body, what you will wear. Is not life more than food, and the body more than clothes?"* Jesus goes on to give an example. If God makes sure that even the sparrows have what they need, he's going to make sure that we also have the things that we need. Whether or not the plumber turns up to fix the washing machine on time, God will still make sure that we're looked after. I'm not saying it's wrong to pray about something so specific, but God's focus is on making sure that we're protected.

I never heard the sermon, but I know one of my friends talked about someone who preached on Philippians 4:19 *"And my God will meet all your needs according to the riches of his glory in Christ Jesus"*. According to the riches of His glory! The preacher said that we 'need' food. We 'need' water. We 'need' clothing. We 'need' medical treatment. And, because we live in a relatively cold country, we 'need' a roof over our head. God will meet all our needs...

The point wasn't that God doesn't give us more than that. I don't 'need' a laptop, except that if I'm going to write this book and hopefully help people by doing so, I 'need' a laptop to be able to follow what I believe I should be doing right now.

The point was that, in this country, we generally don't need to worry about such things. That sermon was preached in the 1990s, and I know that food poverty and energy prices are bigger problems now than they were back then, but God does promise His faithfulness. It may be that through food banks we are part of the solution to providing those things for others, or that our church family helps to ensure that we have what we need. That's still God meeting needs, He's just sending one of us as a messenger!

What we should get from those situations is a sense of freedom. Because we know our actual needs are always met, and because we know that God provides us with abundantly more than we actually need, that question of having faith in whether we'll actually see the plumber on time becomes less important. It's interesting though that when other people have relied upon me for something, and I can't afford to be late because of the impact it will have upon someone else, I've found that in those times prayers seem to be answered about the specific things. Just my experience, or a spiritual point about how God goes about helping? He helps us to be able to do the things that we need to be able to do. As for the washing machine? Well, hopefully it will get fixed soon, but it doesn't really matter. When we understand that it doesn't really matter, that's when the whole question of faith starts to get a lot easier.

If we have faith in the 'wrong' things...

And God doesn't provide that thing...

Then we start to think that faith isn't working...

Our faith gradually erodes...

We lose confidence that God will help...

Then it seems like God is further and further away...

We question the nature of faith...

...and then when a situation comes along where we should absolutely be praying in faith, we find ourselves with doubts.

There's nothing wrong with asking God for anything. He is our father. We can approach him at any time. 1 John 5:14-15 puts it like this:

"This is the confidence we have in approaching God: that if we ask anything according to his will, he hears us. And if we know that he hears us - whatever we ask - we know that we have what we asked of him."

The phrase 'according to His will' is the point here. When our prayers and requests are within His plan, they will be granted. When we go outside His plan and ask for things which we 'want', the answer to that prayer might be 'yes'. It also might be 'no', or it might be 'not yet'. That's perfectly okay, and if we understand that, it won't keep chipping away at our faith and eroding it. Waiting is never easy, just like being given the answer 'no' isn't easy. There's nothing wrong with asking the question, but if we become fixated on those things we start to get away from what we should be focusing on.

Prayer is about much more than requests. God gives us a template for prayer in the Lord's Prayer. Remember that He is our father, that He is in heaven and that His name is higher than any other. Now, our mind is in the right place. We pray for His kingdom to be established - not just in heaven, but right here on this earth. Where His kingdom comes first, the world works better. We pray that His will would be done, again on the earth just like in heaven. If His will is perfect in heaven, we can say the same right here.

We ask for Him to give us our daily bread: the things we need to sustain us through the day. To meet our needs, knowing that He will always fulfil His promises. We ask for forgiveness of our sins (how easy it is to forget that one!), and we pay that forward by also forgiving those who sin against us. We ask for His protection from being tempted, and to keep us well away from things that are evil. Because we know that God has the power and the glory, and that lasts forever. Amen!

There really isn't much about ourselves in the Lord's Prayer. If we're finding praying in faith difficult, sometimes that can be because we're praying for the wrong things.

Let's take a hypothetical situation. You're depressed. You've tried to pray but (remember that 'feelings' don't always represent 'reality') it just feels like God is so far away. It feels like praying isn't helping. You're not necessarily sure what exactly it is that you want to pray about. You speak to some of your Christian friends, and they encourage you to 'pray through it'. Prayer can't ever be bad advice, in itself. The problem can be that your friends maybe are defaulting to an obvious suggestion (I mean, obviously, prayer has definitely been one of the first things on your list to do when struggling) without really listening to what it is that is causing you to struggle. If someone doesn't understand the nature of depression (or honestly, the nature of a number of other things which could be happening), then 'you should pray' can be an easy default comment to make. It feels like a very spiritual, Christian thing to say.

I repeat: not bad advice in itself. Prayer is a good thing. Prayer is important. If you're caring for someone with depression, they're needing something more than a simple suggestion of prayer. Supporting people through depression requires something more. It means you need to get alongside them, love them, be there with them. It means you need to spend significant time with them, offering a helping hand when needed both emotionally and practically. And prayer? Yes! Spend time with them in prayer: it's not something that they need to do on their own (what message is that sending to someone who feels that they're not being understood?) but something that you can do together with them as a key part of the whole process of caring.

Eliphaz, Bildad, and Zophar were Job's friends. They got some things right. They spent time with him. They stayed with him for a whole week. When Job cried, they cried with him. So far, so good. That's the easy part. The first week of caring for someone in a time like that is tiring. Then what about the second, third, fourth weeks? What when you can't quite 'see' the progress after a couple of months? Do *you* still have faith when caring for your depressed friend?

What's where Eliphaz, Bildad, and Zophar went wrong. After a while, I get a sense that they were frustrated. They didn't have all the answers, and so they started to blame Job. Remember Chapter 2? Depression is not a sin. It's easy to start to get irritated. Job's friends just assumed that Job must be sinning 'somehow'. Why would Job be going through all this if it wasn't his fault in some way? There's a modern word 'victim-blaming' which sums up how things can be: if we blame people who are depressed because they are depressed, no wonder those people find it difficult to trust us. It's a bit like prayers for healing: in the Bible, it tells us to 'lay on hands' and pray for the sick. We're told that *"the prayer offered in faith will make the sick person well"* (James 5:16). I haven't heard this said for a few years, thankfully, but I remember many examples of people praying. The sick person did not recover instantly, and so they blamed a 'lack of faith' of the sick person rather than the person doing the praying. It was the polar opposite of James 5 (if you're praying for someone, the question is your faith). And, of course, there is a question as to the circumstances in which it is God's will for divine healing to take place. That's a whole different can of worms. The problem of 'blaming the person you're praying for' is much rarer these days, but it's quite easy to fall into the same trap as Job's friends. Are bad things happening as a result of some 'unconfessed sin' in your life? That's usually pretty shoddy friendship (sin *can* lead to depression on occasion I suppose, but it really shouldn't be the usual thought process when providing support to a friend who's broken) because it starts blaming the person who's already struggling with low self-esteem. The worst thing is that they might start to believe that they're actually to blame, when they're not.

God was not at all pleased with Job's friends. They should have remained supportive, but instead they undermined him. Worse still, by doing so they effectively bad-mouthed God as well:

"After the Lord had said these things to Job, he said to Eliphaz the Temanite, "I am angry with you and your two friends, because you have not spoken the truth about me, as my servant Job has." - Job 42:7

Don't be like Job's friends. There is a better model, supporting each other through times of trial and difficulty. It's found in Ecclesiastes 4:9-12:

"Two are better than one, because they have a good return for their labour: If either of them falls down, one can help the other up. But pity anyone who falls and has no one to help them up. Also, if two lie down together, they will keep warm. But how can one keep warm alone? Though one may be overpowered, two can defend themselves. A cord of three strands is not quickly broken."

That's the kind of friend you should be. We all fall down, from time to time. We need a helping hand when that happens. Such things work better when, in fact, we offer each other that hand. Remember that we're supposed to be imitators of God (Ephesians 5)? Well Psalm 40 tells us that God *"lifted me out of the slimy pit, out of the mud and mire; he set my feet on a rock and gave me a firm place to stand"*.

Or, to put it another way, **we don't ask why someone is stuck in the slimy pit. We help them out of it!**

Once they're safe and sound, it might *then* be appropriate to chat about ways to avoid falling back into the same pit. That's a challenge, because people often only want to talk about pits when they're stuck in one. They might jump right back into the pit, and then it becomes a revolving door. Longer-term strategies become more important than the short-term pit, but that's a much more complex topic.

Chapter 11 - Raise a Hallelujah

"I'm gonna sing, in the middle of the storm. Louder and louder, you're gonna hear my praises roar. Up from the ashes, hope will arise. Death is defeated, the King is alive!" - Raise a Hallelujah, Bethel Music

Yes, I am quoting a song by Bethel Music and I'm not going to apologise for doing so. I've seen some fairly harsh videos criticising them online for some of the ways they do things, accusing them of basically being heretical. The bottom line though is that they believe the key components of the Gospel, they are clearly saved, and I'm not going to refuse to sing their songs when there is obviously a 'good fruit' from them.

There's something about worship. It's a vital component of being a Christian, just like prayer is. Luke 19:37-40 says this:

"When he came near the place where the road goes down the Mount of Olives, the whole crowd of disciples began joyfully to praise God in loud voices for all the miracles they had seen: "Blessed is the king who comes in the name of the Lord! Peace in heaven and glory in the highest!"

Some of the Pharisees in the crowd said to Jesus, "Teacher, rebuke your disciples!" "I tell you," he replied, "if they keep quiet, the stones will cry out.""

God must be praised. But think about it - from whose perspective is that true? In my opinion, God does not 'need' us to praise Him (God is perfect, not egotist) but the real 'need' for praise is because a) it is true, and something of such magnitude that is true should be said, and b) because there is something about praising God which is healthy for us to do because it fixes our eyes in the right direction spiritually.

In this chapter, we're going to talk about that second reason that worship is healthy. It helps us when we worship God. We talked already about prayer, but there is in fact some overlap between prayer and worship. They're not totally different things. Remember how the Lord's Prayer begins? By focusing on God and His qualities. In one sense the first couple of lines can be seen as worship, which then leads to prayer. Indeed, in church services, how often does the worship leader or the person leading the service move seamlessly from a time of worship to a time of prayer? It happens a lot because of that synergy between the two: when we are worshipping God, it places us in the right mindset to be able to pray effectively for the right things. Worship can often be overlooked outside a church service on Sunday mornings. Think about it: most churches will organise 'prayer meetings' either as regular events or special evenings. Some take part in a '24 hours of prayer' session. If you have a small group (Connect Group, Life Group, etc), prayer is likely part of every single session. All very good things to do. How often do churches have a special 'worship evening' in the same way that they do 'prayer evenings'? I feel that in some churches (and that is a comment to The Church as a whole across this nation, not a criticism of any individual church - don't ever take my words as critical in that way), worship needs to be more prominent in what we do.

This leads me to a controversial opinion, but one which I believe in general will help us to deal with depression. I believe our first thought should be 'worship', and our second thought should be 'prayer' when we're helping someone through a time of depression. When you're depressed, it may be most helpful to put some worship music on. If you're caring for someone who's depressed, there can be times when you might want to just spend some time together in worship (context is important here, read the situation first!).

Test what I say here. I understand if you disagree. My reasoning is this: when we worship God, we stop focusing upon our own feelings. Instead we start to focus on things which *we know to be true*: we remind ourselves of how amazing God is. Our focus moves away from the problems we're currently facing, and our own mood. It moves towards those eternal truths. Remember that the Psalms were originally intended to be sung. Throughout the Psalms, we see examples of this: the 'lifting out of the slimy pit' that we saw at the end of the last chapter is an example.

Psalm 30:11-12 says "*You turned my wailing into dancing; you removed my sackcloth and clothed me with joy, that my heart may sing your praises and not be silent. Lord my God, I will praise you forever*". I'm sure we could find dozens of examples throughout the Psalms of this same principle. Psalm 42:5 asks "*Why, my soul, are you downcast? Why so disturbed within me?*

Put your hope in God, for I will yet praise him, my Saviour and my God." Even in a time when we are downcast (or depressed), the solution proposed by the Psalmists is to praise God. As we do so, we begin to find that we are lifted up. Psalm 42 was written by the Sons of Korah. A modern group of musicians used 'Sons of Korah' as their band name and have put many of the Psalms to music. It might be worth checking them out on YouTube, not just out of general curiosity but because I think it starts to give an interesting flavour of the original meaning of the Psalms and because you might find it to be quite 'therapeutic' to play some of them when feeling depressed. I don't like being too prescriptive because every human is different, and depression affects people differently so the best ways to help are different, but I feel this principle of praise is mentioned so often in the BIble that we should take it very seriously.

Leila Grandemange wrote about "How I overcame depression and anxiety through praise and worship":

"Years ago, I didn't know all this. Praising God was mostly for sunny days. That's when it seemed easy to sing worship songs, give thanks, and declare, "God is good!"

But then, God took me through a very dark and stormy valley where I struggled daily with emotional and physical pain. Suddenly, it felt almost impossible to sing God's praise. But I still cried to him for help.

Some days, the emotional and physical pain seemed too much to bear. Feelings of hopelessness plagued me while struggling with anxiety and depression. I also struggled to eat and became horribly thin. My family was so worried and helped the best they could. I often became teary and complained to God, and even grappled with doubts wondering if he truly loved me.

It took many months trudging through the valley of despair to understand that hope is birthed not only by crying to God for help, but also through praise and worship. In other words, we not only pray, "Dear God, please help me, heal me, deliver me..." We also declare and celebrate his goodness and love through song or by whatever means possible, even though things don't seem to be going our way.

She describes her personal journey as follows:

- *Worship music played almost non-stop in my house.*
- *I sang God's praise even when my body ached and my mind felt weary.*
- *I lifted my arms to heaven while singing, even though my heart was heavy.*
- *I prayed, talking to God about my troubles throughout the day, even though I wondered if he was listening.*
- *I trusted in his promises, putting one foot in front of the other, even though I felt afraid.*
- *I gave thanks to God in my pain, even when I didn't feel thankful.*
- *I worshiped and praised him, while clinging to the promise that God loved me and was always with me.*

Taken from LeilaGrandemange.com, © Leila Grandemange.

Notice how vital worship became in that healing process from depression. Never underestimate the power of praising God! There is a hope, an indescribable hope, which comes from God. As we worship Him, as we draw closer to Him, that hope starts to become more real. Where negative feelings and the spiritual reality are in conflict, worship helps to realign the two and bring our feelings back into line with the truth of God's Word.

Chapter 12 - A higher purpose

"Just as a body, though one, has many parts, but all its many parts form one body, so it is with Christ"

- 1 Corinthians 12:12

I've touched on this already, but there is a sense of 'calling' about being a Christian. You may not feel that you have been specifically called to a particular ministry (and that's perfectly okay). But God does give us spiritual gifts. If you grew up in a Pentecostal background, you might be used to hearing more about the gifts of tongues and prophecy. But in Isaiah, Romans and 1 Corinthians we get much more:

Isaiah 11:2 "The Spirit of the Lord will rest on him - the Spirit of wisdom and of understanding, the Spirit of counsel and of might, the Spirit of the knowledge and fear of the Lord"

Romans 12:6-8 "We have different gifts, according to the grace given to each of us. If your gift is prophesying, then prophesy in accordance with your faith; if it is serving, then serve; if it is teaching, then teach; if it is to encourage, then give encouragement; if it is giving, then give generously; if it is to lead, do it diligently; if it is to show mercy, do it cheerfully."

1 Corinthians 12:8-11 "To one there is given through the Spirit a message of wisdom, to another a message of knowledge by means of the same Spirit, to another faith by the same Spirit, to another gifts of healing by that one Spirit, to another miraculous powers, to another prophecy, to another distinguishing between spirits, to another speaking in different kinds of tongues, and to still another the interpretation of tongues. All these are the work of one and the same Spirit, and he distributes them to each one, just as he determines."

1 Corinthians 12: 27-31 "Now you are the body of Christ, and each one of you is a part of it. And God has placed in the church first of all apostles, second prophets, third teachers, then miracles, then gifts of healing, of helping, of guidance, and of different kinds of tongues. Are all apostles? Are all prophets? Are all teachers? Do all work miracles? Do all have gifts of healing? Do all speak in tongues? Do all interpret? Now eagerly desire the greater gifts."

The spiritual gifts are so much broader than tongues and prophecy. The gift of 'wisdom', the gift of 'teaching' and the gift of 'guidance' are absolutely fundamental to the day-to-day functioning of the church. The idea is that across the whole body of the church, these gifts should be in evidence. Just as the body has many parts (1 Corinthians 12:12), so too does the church. If your role is to be an arm, you shouldn't wish that you were a foot instead! The body needs all its parts to work together.

Even the (rather long) lists of spiritual gifts given here aren't necessarily intended to be exhaustive. The fact that we have different lists in different passages suggests that we're being given examples, rather than being told that every gift is listed here. I do very strongly feel that when you understand your 'role' within the Body of Christ, it helps with a broader sense of purpose in your life. Remember Proverbs 29:18, where we're told that without vision the people would perish? Having vision and purpose provides a structure.

How many people have the gift of administration, for example? Now when I use that word, it's the same as the one translated 'guidance' in the NIV. The Greek word kubernēsis means both: it is used for the pilot of a ship in Acts 27, and is used similarly in the [Greek translation of the] Old Testament. It has a different connotation to the pastor of a church. Perhaps we should think of the word as the 'person who makes everything run smoothly behind the scenes and usually doesn't get enough credit for doing so'. I'm sure you can think of such people in your own church. They are a blessing, and perhaps that is what you're supposed to do.

Part of the role of the Church is to develop and equip its members: Ephesians 4:11-13 says that He *"gave the apostles, the prophets, the evangelists, the pastors and teachers, to equip his people for works of service, so that the body of Christ may be built up until we all reach unity in the faith and in the knowledge of the Son of God and become mature, attaining to the whole measure of the fullness of Christ"*. In other words, the so-called ministry gifts aren't just about standing at the front of church and 'leading' (although people with those gifts may do that). There is also a practical sense in which, if you have those gifts, it's your job to help others to develop their own gifts. As we do that, other people develop into their own roles and that's where the 'measure of the fullness of Christ' comes in. So where do you fit into all that? Well, it depends very much on you - but that's probably a great area to pray into. Once you understand where you 'fit' within the Church (capital C, not necessarily the church you attend on a Sunday), you'll also have a greater sense of purpose and vision in your life. Having such a sense of purpose is a huge help when it comes to fighting depression: how can you feel depressed when you've got a strong sense of belonging and an understanding that you're on a mission which God Himself has sent you on? Note that I talk about the Church as a whole, because for some people your main 'calling' or 'spiritual job' might be within the body of Christ but outside the church structure. I know many people who work in Christian ministries and charities, whether voluntarily or as a full-time job, which are only tangentially connected to the church they attend on a Sunday.

This is a challenge, as well, to those who are supporting another Christian who has depression - or, indeed, other mental health issues. Do 'we' in the see the person in church who suffers from depression or anxiety as being somehow just someone to be cared for, and not as a functioning part of the body?

Let's explain that with an analogy. What do you do if you've got 'pins and needles' in your leg? You get up and you exercise the leg to get the blood flowing and the circulation moving again. Remember that the person with mental health issues is every bit as much a part of the church body as a leg is part of yours: it's important that the leg actually acts as a leg!

In his book 'What is life without my love?', Ian Jennings talks about the concept of a 'big plan' even in the deepest of grief:

"It is sometimes hard to shake the thought that there is no 'big plan' and that life is just a series of random events. The concept of the 'big plan' can feel like a bad joke in poor taste when all your careful plans have crumbled into dust. It may be hard to find purpose. Yet as we still the turbulence of our hearts and invite God to calm our anxious thoughts, He will prompt us to an awareness that we are still part of His greater plan."

Yet that sense of purpose is there too. Ian points out that in Isaiah 30:21, we have a promise that God will be with us guiding us through the process of getting back on our feet:

"Whether you turn to the right or to the left, your ears will hear a voice behind you, saying, "This is the way; walk in it."

Finally, he reminds us of Jeremiah 29:11: *"For I know the plans I have for you," declares the Lord, "plans to prosper you and not to harm you, plans to give you hope and a future."*

It may be, though, that we have to wait a while before plans become evident. Look back at the previous verse, Jeremiah 29:10, for the context: the Israelites had to wait for seventy years before the promises in verse 11 actually happened. Yes, God does have a plan for you. Yes, He will guide you. His word is a 'lamp' to your feet (Psalm 119:105). There may be a time of waiting, but we will get there in the end.

- Don't downplay God's plans for our life, even if we have to wait.
- Remember that we have a royal command. We are on the King's business together.
- That should give us the positivity and vision that we need.

Chapter 13 - Practical advice

"Finally, brothers and sisters, whatever is true, whatever is noble, whatever is right, whatever is pure, whatever is lovely, whatever is admirable - if anything is excellent or praiseworthy - think about such things." - Philippians 4:8

We've covered a lot of the 'spiritual' side of dealing with depression, but what should we be doing on a day-to-day basis? We know that the world will give us many suggestions about how to look after ourselves. Some of them are good, some of them are outright dangerous, and others have it half-right. Don't forget, however good the advice might be, God should be at the centre of your decision-making process.

What the world says...

If you're suffering from depression, you need to take antidepressant medication to feel better.

What a Christian should actually do...

God has provided us with doctors and nurses, trained medical professionals, for a reason. There are many other things you should try first before medication, but if (after prayer and consultation with your doctor) it seems like medication is appropriate for you, that's okay!

What the world says...

You need to get therapy!

What a Christian should actually do...

Don't forget that as a Christian, speaking with other Christians is likely to help more because they will understand your world-view far better. So-called 'talking therapies' can help, but it's better if they're also grounded in your Christian faith. If therapy is needed, then where possible try to speak with a Christian therapist. A lot of this depends on money: therapy on the NHS can have waiting lists and very little choice, whereas private counsellors and therapists cost money but you can certainly find a Christian.

Irrespective of whether or not you feel that therapy is right for you, again after prayer and consultation with your doctor, it's still important to spend time speaking with your church leaders and Christian friends. Worshipping God together, enjoying a meal together and being honest about how you feel, and of course praying together, all can have a 'therapeutic' effect too!

What the world says...

You need to learn to love yourself. Be kind to yourself and spend lots of time on self-care. Run a scented bath, relax, enjoy! Put yourself first.

What a Christian should actually do...

All of those practical things are good to do - but, remember that loving yourself can flow from God's love for you. Definitely take good care of yourself, but remember that Philippians 2: 3-4 tells us *"Do nothing out of selfish ambition or vain conceit, but in humility consider others better than yourselves. Each of you should look not only to your own interests, but also to the interests of others"*. In other words, there's a balance to be struck. Don't allow yourself to become so inward-looking and focused on 'feeling good' that you neglect those around you. On the other hand, remember that you are the 'apple of God's eye' and His 'special possession', so it's certainly a good idea to make sure you look after yourself!

What the world says...

You need a break from everything. Lighten up a bit! Have some casual sex, drink alcohol or take drugs. Or just eat a whole tub of chocolate ice cream. You'll soon forget why you were depressed in the first place.

What a Christian should actually do...

Um, let's just say 'not that'. Very, very bad advice. Well, except the chocolate ice cream. Nothing wrong with that, in moderation. But in 1 Corinthians 6:19-20, Paul reminds us of how important our bodies are to God:

"Do you not know that your bodies are temples of the Holy Spirit, who is in you, whom you have received from God? You are not your own; you were bought at a price. Therefore honor God with your bodies."

You know how you see scams online that seem too good to be true, and they probably are too good to be true? In a similar way, people are trying to 'sell' you a fake dream. The idea that alcohol will cure it is nonsense. You may distract yourself for a short time, but if you're not dealing with the problem you just end up creating a cycle of using alcohol as a crutch. That isn't going to help at all. In the same way, casual sex causes spiritual problems. The spiritual bond created during such an intimate time doesn't work well with the word 'casual'. It has long-term damaging effects.

Having said all of that, there can be a value in less-drastic distraction techniques. Worship is obviously a good 'distraction' because it's more than just a distraction, but on a 'human' level if you head out to the cinema and watch a film with your friends to make sure you get out of the house and have some fun, that might be useful too.

What the world says...

Don't forgive those who hurt you!

What a Christian should actually do...

Unforgiveness means that you're carrying bitterness around in your heart. How will that help you? If anything, it gets in the way. Emotional baggage can weigh heavily on you. Forgiveness lightens that load because it helps you along the road to letting that baggage go. Forgiveness is also something that God tells us to do, just as much for our benefit as for other people's.

It's a command. Not just once, but 'seventy times seven times' (Matthew 18:22). Forgiveness should be a way of life for us as Christians, because we know that God first forgave us.

What if my question isn't covered here?

There are many more things which the world will try to tell us. I couldn't possibly cover all of them at once, so instead we should just think about the general principles. First, test things: does it make sense according to the Word of God? Second, pray about it. If you're not sure, then the best person to ask is God Himself. And third, talk to mature Christians about it. Listen to their advice and weigh it carefully. Then, decide what you want to do.

Where else can I get support from?

1. If you are concerned for your immediate safety (planning to seriously hurt yourself or others), then you need to either go to A&E or call 999.

2. The National Christian Helpline on 0300 111 0101 is open from 9am to midnight, run by Premier [Christian Radio].

3. The UCB Christian Helpline can be contacted on 01782 36 3000, 9am to 10pm Monday to Friday and 10am to 6pm on Saturdays. It is a prayer support line, not a counselling service.

4. The online Christian service chatnow.org allows you to chat online to a

Christian anonymously, 24 hours a day. They also have some useful resources on their site.

5. If you need to speak to someone at any time of day (not a Christian service) then you can contact the Samaritans: 116 123.

6. If you need to find a Christian counsellor, try the Association of Christian Counsellors: www.acc-uk.org. Do be aware, though, that it's important to check that the therapist concerned actually holds to the kind of belief that we would consider to be Christian. Due diligence is important: do they believe the Bible to be the literal, accurate Word of God? Are they going to make sure that God is at the centre of things and help you to recover?

Having said all of the above, I do really believe that friends, family and your church are vital on a day-to-day basis. People who know you and truly love you can make a very special kind of difference in your life.

Don't ever forget God. He can and does help. He cares in ways we can barely even begin to understand. I wish you all the best with your battle against depression, and/or in supporting others. That ultimately goes back to God, and the words in Ephesians 3:20-21 remind us of His power. Amen!

"Now to him who is able to do immeasurably more than all we ask or imagine, according to his power that is at work within us, to him be glory in the church and in Christ Jesus throughout all generations, for ever and ever! Amen."